just
one
thing

just one thing

How simple changes can transform your life

DR MICHAEL MOSLEY

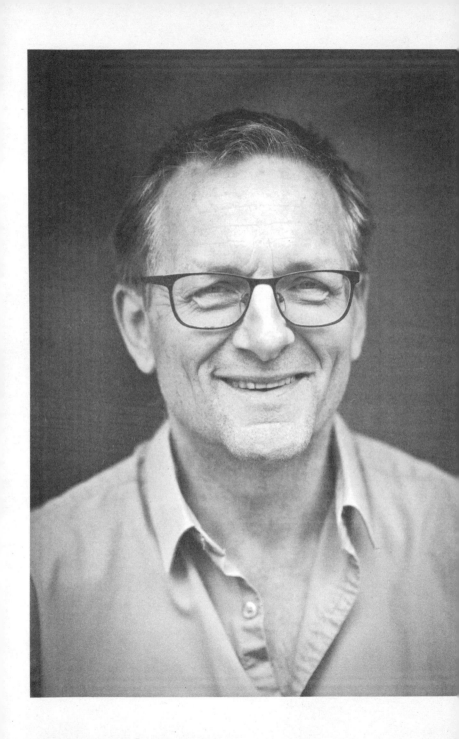

INTRODUCTION

Although I originally trained as a doctor, I have spent most of my long and enjoyable career as a science journalist and TV presenter. This has enabled me to cover a lot of different subjects, but in recent years I have focused on exploring the science behind the many and varied health claims that I have come across. And, of course, trying things out on myself. I've done some pretty crazy things in my time, including infecting myself with parasites, getting leeched, injecting my face with some of my own blood and swallowing a tiny camera so I could watch the workings of my gut. But it was in 2012, when I discovered that I had type 2 diabetes, that I got really serious about wanting to understand the drivers of mental and physical health.

Discovering I had type 2 diabetes led to me making a programme called 'Eat, Fast and Live Longer', during which I came across research showing the benefits of intermittent fasting. Over the course of eight weeks, I lost 9kg by doing a form of intermittent fasting which I called the 5:2 diet, and this enabled me to get my blood sugars back to normal, without medication. That, in turn, led me to write, with Mimi Spencer, *The Fast Diet*, which became an international bestseller, then to write more books (often with my wife Clare, who is a GP and bestselling recipe book writer), covering subjects ranging from weight loss and sleep, to exercise and ways to improve gut health.

Then, in 2021, during the Covid lockdown, I did something very different. I made my first ever podcast series. It was for BBC Sounds and Radio 4 and it was called Just One Thing. Setting up a recording studio in my home during lockdown was a challenge, but as I will show you, trying out new things is really good for your brain (see page 178), particularly an ageing brain like mine, and I loved doing it.

The idea of the podcast is simple: each 15-minute episode introduces Just One Thing you can do to improve your health. The series (which is ongoing) is full of quirky, fun and sometimes bizarre facts, and making it gives me the chance to interview eminent, and often very entertaining, scientists who are leaders in their field. In each episode we find a brave volunteer to give the thing a test run, and, of course, I also give it a go (if you listen to one of the early podcasts you'll hear me yelping at my first blast of a cold shower. See page 24 for more on the science behind cold water immersion).

I was blessed with a very talented team, who made it happen and helped ensure it became a real hit. A big part of the appeal of Just One Thing is its simplicity, and I think that is also what makes it such a great way to turn good intentions into sustainable habits.

After all, most of us recognise the importance of keeping to a healthy weight, eating well, doing regular exercise, reducing stress and getting a good night's sleep. So what stops us? Well, firstly we are bombarded on a daily basis by a lot of vague and often conflicting advice in newspapers, TV and social media: drink coffee, don't drink coffee, cut down on fat, eat more fat, get out in the sun, cover up with sunscreen, exercise slowly or step up the pace…who to believe?

Then there is the problem of putting good advice into practice, of creating a new healthy habit and sticking to it. Many of us start off each New Year resolved to be healthier and more active, but within a month or so most of us have returned to our previous way of life. I don't think this is because we are inherently lazy or weak-willed – it is because we haven't created the environment where a new habit will stick. If you genuinely want to change then here are 10 rules, based on science, which I have found useful:

1. MAKE IT SIMPLE. The rationale behind Just One Thing is that you don't have to do a major overhaul of your life; these are things you can easily build into your routine. Small changes really can yield big benefits in terms of better mood, improved sleep, a sharper brain and reduced disease risk.

2. BE REALISTIC. Although I am going to try to excite you about all the benefits that come from doing lots of Just One Things, begin by doing what you think you can manage. Start small and build from there. That, after all, is the great advantage of this approach. You can always add in Just One More Thing later.

3. CREATE A TRIGGER. You are much more likely to do something if it is attached to an activity you are already doing. As you will see in the next chapter, I do my resistance exercises straight after I get out of bed because I know if I don't do them then I will never do them. I use 'getting out of bed' (which I have to do every day) as a trigger for these exercises. You can use 'having a meal' as a trigger to drink a large glass of water and that way you ensure that you drink enough water during the day (see page 58 for the multiple benefits of doing that) or leaving a notepad and pen beside your bed as a trigger-reminder for journalling (see page 196 for the benefits of 'counting your blessings'). I practise standing on one leg while brushing my teeth, as a way of improving my balance (see page 70) because I know I will never go to regular yoga classes, but I do have to brush my teeth twice a day, so that seemed more realistic. You will come across lots more 'triggers' as you go through the book.

4. KNOW WHY YOU ARE DOING IT. I strongly believe that if you really understand what the benefits are, and can remind yourself of them when the temptation to give up is strong, then you are much more likely to stick to something. That's why this book contains lots of interviews with leading scientists, as well as references to scientific studies, which are easy to look up online. I want you to be convinced that these things are worth doing and persisting with. I also want you to tailor them to your own requirements.

5. STICK WITH IT FOR AT LEAST A MONTH. There is a widely held belief that you can introduce a new habit in 21 days. This is almost certainly untrue. A study published in the *European Journal of Social Psychology* concluded that it took anywhere between 18 and 254 days to ingrain a new habit, so stick with it!

6. TRY TO DISPLACE BAD HABITS WITH GOOD ONES. Many bad habits are deeply ingrained and may be almost impossible to shake. What you can do is try to displace them with better habits. This takes time and persistence.

7. TRY TO DO IT DAILY. Establishing a new habit is mainly about consistency and frequency. Although it is important to know why you are doing something, it is even more important to actually do it and do it on a regular basis. A lot of the things you will come across in this book can be done daily and even sometimes more than once a day. I have also tried to keep them short, as the shorter something is, the more likely you are to stick to it.

8. INVOLVE A FRIEND OR LOVED ONE. One of the main reasons why people pay for personal exercise trainers is that they feel they need someone around to make them do it – it's not that they don't know what to do. Doing a thing with a friend or loved one not only makes you more accountable; it can also make it more fun. Clare and I do a lot of things together, ranging from early-morning workouts to making fermented foods (see page 64), because we have a shared interest in healthy living and because it keeps us motivated. A good reason to get a dog (another thing I should probably have added to the list), apart from the love and companionship, is that dog owners are far more likely to go for walks. In fact, a study carried out in the UK of nearly 700 people, a mix of dog owners and non-dog owners, found those with a four-legged friend were four times more likely to hit the widely recommended health target of 150 minutes per week of moderately vigorous exercise (see page 44). We have a King Charles called Tari, who is over 10 years old, but who still gets incredibly excited every time she even thinks a walk is in the offing. Her joy is a powerful incentive for me to go.

9. BE KIND TO YOURSELF. If you have found a thing that you really like the look of, but just can't stick to it, then perhaps it is not right for you. Don't beat yourself up: accept that this may not be the moment in your life when it works for you. Take a look through the book and see what else appeals to you.

10. KEEP A RECORD. As I pointed out earlier, I like self-experimenting, which means that I also like monitoring change. Try noting down some of your health markers and measurements – such as your weight, your waist, your heart rate, your blood pressure (equipment for this can be bought in a chemist or online) or your blood sugars (ditto). You may find it helpful to invest in a tracker. Keeping a record will show you how far you have come.

In summary: this book is all about quick and simple scientifically proven ways to improve health and wellbeing in a sustainable way. No one is expecting you to do all of them, or even more than one! Just pick and choose what works for you. The advantage of aiming for bite-sized goals is that they will get you thinking, 'OK, I could manage that', and then, hopefully, you might find you are enjoying the activity and end up tagging it on to your life.

choosing your thing

I am so convinced of the benefits of the Just One Things I write about in this book that many of them now form a part of my daily routine. I've chosen to fan out my favourite 30 things across a typical day so you can see how they might fit into your life. There is a wealth of things to choose from; and obviously I don't want you to try them all at once! But I hope you find yourself tempted to start by trying one or two, and be encouraged by the benefits they bring.

For some of the things, the timing is important. A walk has added benefits when you get outside in the early-morning light; coffee is best drunk a couple of hours after you've woken up; you'll get more vitamin D from a blast of sunshine in the middle of the day; and a hot bath works best as part of a snooze-inducing, wind-down routine in the evening, not the morning. But the rest? Mix them up as much of you like. In fact, a few things – such as drinking water, singing, standing up, taking a break and deep breathing – can be happily peppered at intervals throughout your day.

The first thing on my daily list is always 'intelligent exercises' (squats and press-ups) because I know I'll never get around to them if I leave them until later; likewise, I really enjoy a spoonful of sauerkraut with my breakfast omelette. But that's me. You might like the idea of starting the day with a bit of mindful meditation and enjoying fermented foods with your lunch or dinner instead. It's good to know that breaking into song will be just as beneficial whatever time of day the urge strikes.

So flick through the book, pick one new thing you want to try and give it a go. Once you've made that a habitual part of your life, browse the book again and see if there's another you fancy trying.

Good luck! Michael

EARLY MORNING
Intelligent exercises
Cold shower
Sing
Meditate
Early-morning walk

BREAKFAST
Change your mealtimes
Drink water
Eat some bacteria
Stand on one leg
Drink coffee

MID-MORNING
Take a break
Deep breaths
Exercise less, but more often
Eccentric exercise
Think yourself stronger

LUNCHTIME
Enjoy oily fish
Eat beetroot
An apple a day
Get some sun
Take a nap

AFTERNOON
Get some house plants
Play video games
Green spaces
Stand up
Eat chocolate

EVENING
Dance
Learn a new skill
Hot bath
Read
Count your blessings

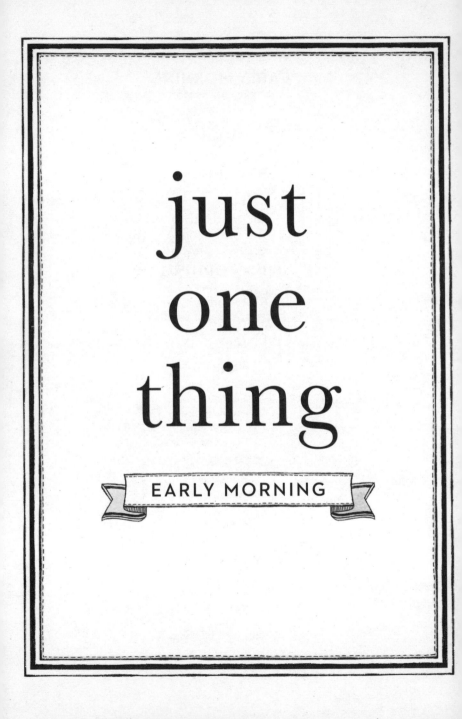

just one
thing

EARLY MORNING

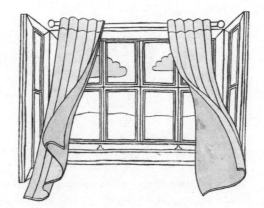

intelligent exercises

How to do it: do a couple of minutes of squats or press-ups every day.

I don't know about you, but I used to find it incredibly easy to sleep through the night. When I was a teenager I slept in a telephone box, a graveyard and even on the platform of a railway station in India. Sadly, getting a good night's sleep is no longer a given. These days I often wake around 3am, roam around the house for a bit, then make my way back to bed when I am feeling tired. What I am trying to do is teach my brain to associate 'bed' with 'sleep' and 'sex' and nothing else. The health benefits of sexual intercourse are many and varied, although this is Just One Thing I haven't really looked into yet. There is, however, another form of exercise that I would heartily recommend and that I do first thing: intelligent exercises.

Whatever my night has been like, I wake up at roughly the same time every morning (around 7am), get out of bed, open the curtains, enjoy the early-morning light, wake Clare (who often grumbles), turn on the radio and together we start doing our first Just One Thing of the day: resistance exercises. I hasten to add that you don't need to do them first thing, but I do think it is really important that you do them at some point in the day.

We all know that doing aerobic exercise (running, swimming, cycling) is good for your heart and lungs, but less than 5 per cent of people regularly do exercises which are specifically targeted at building muscle. And that is tragic because after the age of 30, unless you do something about it, you will start to lose around 5 per cent of your muscle mass for every decade that passes. And you need that muscle, you really do.

Being more muscly not only makes you look good, it improves your posture and reduces your risk of developing back pain. Muscles burn calories, even when you are asleep, and they are also, obviously, essential for keeping you active. So it is vital that you do what you can to build and preserve them. And it is never too late to start.

One of the best ways to build your muscles is to do more resistance exercises. Resistance exercises are any exercises where you use your muscles to lift or pull against resistance. This could involve lifting weights, or using resistance bands, which come in a wide range of sizes and strengths. But I prefer something I can do at home, or when I am on the road, filming, and which doesn't involve any equipment. So instead of weights I do squats and press-ups, where you are using your own body weight to make your muscles work harder. As well as being simple to do, press-ups and squats are some of the best exercises for your heart and brain.

I normally start by doing 30–40 press-ups. That sounds like bragging, which it certainly is, but I have built up to this gradually. What I love about press-ups is that they are a fast and very effective way to build upper body strength. I also like the fact that I can do a lot more than Clare (though she is catching up). The number of press-ups you can do also seems to be a good predictor of heart health.

In a study carried out by researchers from the Harvard School of Public Health, 1000 firemen in their early forties were asked to do as many press-ups as they could in a minute. When the same men were seen 10 years later, it turned out that those who had managed to do 40 or more press-ups in the earlier test were 96 per cent less likely to have had a heart attack than those who managed 10 or fewer. Unfortunately, they didn't do this test with women, but broadly speaking, you would expect a woman to be able to do half as many press-ups, for her age, as a man. A man in his fifties should be able to do 20, a woman at least 10.

As well as press-ups, I do at least 30 squats first thing every morning (squats are where you bend your knees as if you are about to sit on a chair). Squats work the biggest muscles in your body and are probably the best single exercise you can do. As I said, they are not just good for your body but for your brain too.

Damian Bailey is professor of physiology and biochemistry and director of the Neurovascular Research Laboratory at the University of South Wales. He told me that any form of exercise is likely to be good for the brain but they have found that the action of moving your body up and down against resistance (i.e. the squat) seems to be particularly effective at stimulating blood flow to a part of the brain responsible for learning and memory (the hippocampus). Which is why I call this an 'intelligent' exercise.

Doing squats not only provides an increased blood supply but also stimulates the release of a hormone called BDNF (brain-derived neurotrophic factor) which encourages the growth of new brain cells and connections. Think of it as fertiliser for your brain.

'We know that, as we get older, blood flow through the hippocampus tends to decrease, leading to cognitive decline and neurodegeneration in later life, and it is clear that exercise can boost blood supply to the brain, causing the area to grow,' he told me.

'However, our work shows that squats also appear to challenge the brain with an increase and then a decrease in blood flow. This "to and fro" action challenges the inner lining of the arteries which supply blood to the brain, triggering the release of chemicals which trigger brain growth.'

He added, 'We are increasingly aware that it's not just the amount of blood flow through your brain, it is the quality and the intermittency of the flow which optimises the "good molecules" that move into the brain tissue and stimulate new connections and new cells.'

Interestingly, Professor Bailey's work shows squats have a more powerful brain-boosting effect than walking or jogging: 'We have identified that 3–5 minutes of squats three times a week is even more effective in terms of brain health than a brisk 30-minute jog three times a week,' he says. 'It is like a form of interval training for the brain – no huffing and puffing required.'

As a press-ups fan, I was delighted to hear that doing them has a similar effect. 'It is this general action of your head moving up and down, working against gravity, that seems to benefit the brain,' he told me.

And the good news for couch potatoes is that Professor Bailey's research shows people who have rarely exercised still get the brain benefits of squats and press-ups, if they take them up later in life.

So why not see if doing some press-ups and squats is Just One Thing you could get into? The key is to start gradually to avoid injury. If you have an existing back problem or high blood pressure or are frail, talk to your doctor before starting.

Overleaf, I describe how to do them, but if you are in any doubt watch an online video. (If you search for 'NHS strength exercises' you will find quite a few options.) You could, of course, go to a gym and get instructions on how to do them properly.

Clare and I use 'getting out of bed' as our trigger for doing resistance exercises, but you may prefer doing them at other times. A friend of mine uses 'boiling the kettle for a cup of tea' as his trigger to do some squats or press-ups, while another does a few every time she goes to the loo (afterwards, obviously).

Don't worry if early-morning intelligent exercises aren't for you – there are lots of other things you can try that will set you up for the day. Such as having a cold shower.

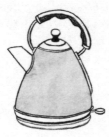

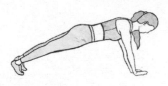

PRESS-UPS

Start with the easiest option, standing facing a wall, your feet firmly planted on the floor, hip width apart, and your arms outstretched, palms on the wall at shoulder height. Now simply bend your arms and, keeping your back and legs straight, let your upper body sink towards the wall; then use your arms to push yourself back again.

You can progress to push-ups off the back of a garden bench, or a work top, and then get down on the floor to perform what is sometimes known as a 'half press-up', where, with your arms straight and your hands directly below your shoulders, you do the same 'push-up' action from your knees, only attempting the full body press-up (keeping your body poker straight and your abdominal muscles sucked in) when knee press-ups feel easy.

SQUATS

With feet shoulder width apart and toes facing forwards, slowly lower your bottom as if you are about to sit on a chair behind you, keeping your tummy tight and your back straight. Then squeeze your buttocks and drive yourself up to standing again.

You can start by resting your hand on a work surface or the back of a chair to help you balance, and gradually increase the depth of the squat as you become more flexible.

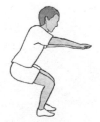

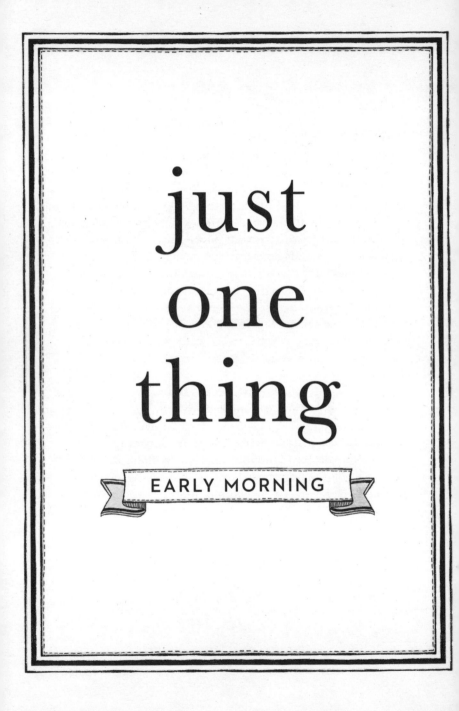

just one thing

EARLY MORNING

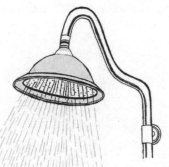

cold shower

How to do it : after your normal warm shower, turn the tap to the coldest setting and breathe slowly and steadily for 10–60 seconds.

I have to confess, when this Just One Thing was first put to me, I was pretty horrified. But if less than a minute of discomfort each day really can help you combat stress and bolster your immune system, it's got to be worth a try, right?

Rather than opt for an immediate cold soaking, I start by getting in a warm shower, washing myself, then turning the hot tap off. The first time I did this it was a real shock. There was lots of shrieking from the bathroom and I was out of there in under 10 seconds. I've got better with practice. These days I'm no longer doing quite as much hyperventilating and jumping from foot to foot, and I can last a minute, even in winter. But I'm still not as calm and controlled as Clare, who seems to be happy to stand serene and silent with icy water pouring down on her head. One of my sons, Daniel, who has been a disciple of Wim Hof, 'The Iceman', since he came across him on YouTube, not only loves a cold shower every morning but swims in the Thames on Christmas Day.

As well as cold showers, cold water swimming is becoming increasingly popular, thanks to claims that it can boost your mood, lower stress, improve your cardiovascular health and strengthen your immune system. So what's going on?

Well, the first time you jump in the sea in winter, or have an icy-cold shower, it will, not surprisingly, trigger a stress response. You will start hyperventilating, your heart rate will shoot up and your body will be flooded with adrenaline. The shock of the cold water sends your circulatory system into overdrive.

But if you keep on doing it, your body will, over time, get used to it. Research has shown that it takes six immersions in cold water to halve our stress response – our heart rate doesn't rise as much, we panic less.

The idea is that repeatedly undergoing the mild stressor of immersion in cold water will help you cope with other stressors as well.

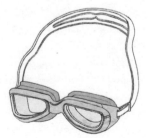

Although much of the research is still in its infancy, Mike Tipton, who is professor of human and applied physiology at the Extreme Environments Laboratory at Portsmouth University, thinks that this cross-adaption could help explain some of the benefits of cold water immersion. He has shown, for example, that exposing people to the stress of cold showers makes them better able to tolerate being at high altitude, and he thinks this cross-coping mechanism might also explain why people who do regular cold water swimming often find it helps their mental health.

'Anecdotal evidence,' he told me, 'is the weakest form of evidence but we know there are literally thousands of people who will tell you that going into cold water has improved their mood and morale. We've done a case study with an individual who had postnatal depression. She went through a cold habituation programme, which involved cold water immersion. She went from being incredibly unhappy to saying she was the happiest she'd been in years. A year later, she's still doing open water swimming, is pretty much drug free and depression free.' This particular case study was published in the *British Medical Journal*.

Learning to cope with the stress of cold water immersion could also explain why having cold showers might help you fight infection. In a large trial, carried out in the Netherlands in the winter months, 3018 volunteers, aged between 18 and 65 and with no previous experience of regular cold showers, were randomly allocated to having a cold shower or a warm shower every morning, for a month. The study found that those who had the cold shower took 30 per cent fewer days off sick from work than the control group.

Finally, cold water immersion appears to have an anti-inflammatory effect, which is important when you consider that so many of the modern conditions that affect us – Alzheimer's, type 2 diabetes, heart disease, depression – have their root in chronic inflammation.

So if you fancy making cold water immersion Just One Thing you'd like to try, how should you go about it? Firstly, it would be a good idea to acclimatise yourself to cold exposure by starting off with brief cold showers. I recommend you begin with a warm shower followed by a 10-second cold shower, and then gradually build up your exposure.

Mercifully, you don't have to spend very long in a cold shower to gain benefits (in fact, staying in too long can be counterproductive). Professor Tipton told me that the important thing is to remain in long enough to get your breathing under control. In the Dutch study they found no particular benefit to staying in longer than a minute.

If you are planning on moving on from showers to cold water swimming, try it with a friend or join a club (there are lots of them out there). And do check with your GP first if you have any underlying health conditions as getting cold really can be a double-edged sword.

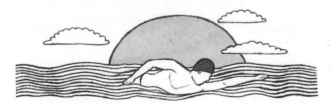

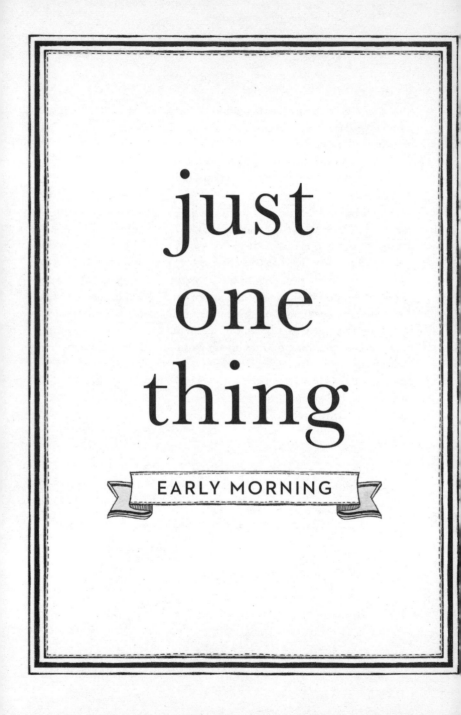

just
one
thing

EARLY MORNING

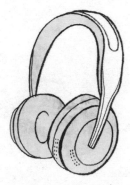

sing

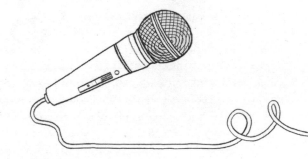

How to do it: sing loudly for five minutes a day.

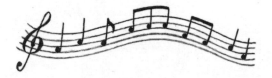

When I am having my cold shower I often start singing, loudly.
Not because I'm any good – I can barely hold a tune – but because
I find it really helps me get through the first, painful 20 seconds
or so. More generally, I would recommend you take up singing, in
the bathroom or anywhere else, because research shows it is a great
way to boost mood, reduce anxiety and even relieve chronic pain.
Also, and most importantly, it is fun.

One way singing makes us feel good and gives us a natural
'high' is by boosting our endocannabinoids. These are chemicals
naturally produced in our bodies that have a very similar structure
to those found in the cannabis plant; in high concentration they
can have mood-boosting effects.

A few years ago, I took part in a study at Nottingham
University, in which we asked a group of middle-aged women,
who sing together as part of the Derbyshire and Nottinghamshire
Rock Choir, to try out a number of different activities to see
which boosted levels of their endocannabinoids the most.

We tested their bloods before and after cycling in a group, singing in a choir, taking part in a dance class and doing a 'boring' activity (the control), which involved sitting and reading a dishwasher instruction manual.

All the activities, apart from reading the instruction manual, had some effect but a 30-minute session of group singing boosted blood levels of endocannabinoids by the most, a whopping 42 per cent (twice as much as cycling!). And, fortunately, you don't have to be good to enjoy the benefits.

Dr Daisy Fancourt is associate professor of psychobiology and epidemiology at University College London. She believes there is something very special about singing: 'It is a behaviour that has been with us for tens of thousands of years and it has always played an important role in human evolution,' she told me. 'Anthropological studies show singing plays a part in group bonding, communication, healing rituals and collective expressions of emotion, and the fact that it occurs in cultures all around the world suggests it has intrinsic benefit for humans.'

The benefits, Dr Fancourt believes, come from the different component parts of singing: there is the pleasure of being immersed in music, the physicality of breathing, plus the fact that it is often a social activity. 'Singing appears to activate so many different systems it can have multiple effects all at once,' she says.

Studies by her team at UCL have found a single session of singing can lead to improvements in mood and measurable reductions in stress and inflammation. Her team have also measured improvements in lung function in people with lung diseases and in memory in people with dementia, as well as notable reductions in blood pressure and muscle tension, and feelings of loneliness. In addition to this, UCL trials have shown that enrolling in singing programmes led to significant reductions in postnatal depression in just a few weeks.

Studies show that the natural endocannabinoid high you get from singing can also help with pain relief. When I was involved in one such study, a volunteer told me he found it better than all the tablets in the world.

So why not give singing a try? Research from the British Academy of Sound Therapy shows singing along to 'positive music' (that means anything that you personally like) for more than five minutes a day is enough to improve your mood. Follow Dr Fancourt's advice, and make singing a daily habit by linking it with another activity, such as having a shower or making your breakfast. Even better, join a choir.

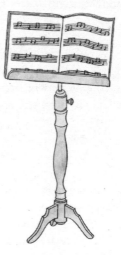

Studies show
that the natural
endocannabinoid
high you get from
singing can also
help with pain relief.
When I was involved
in one such study,
a volunteer told me
he found it better
than all the tablets
in the world.

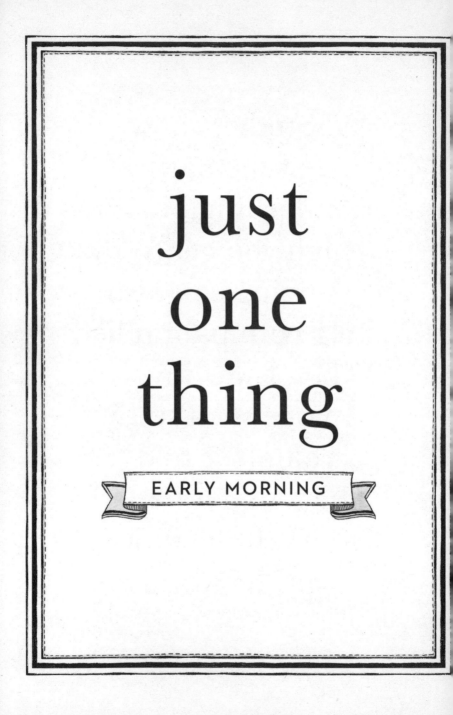

just one thing

EARLY MORNING

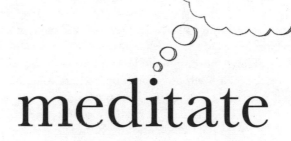

meditate

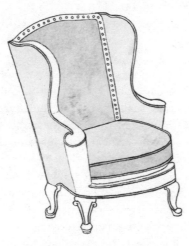

How to do it: practise mindful meditation for 10 minutes every day.

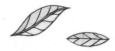

Many of us go through life with self-critical and unhelpful thoughts rattling around inside our heads, each one competing for our attention. These constant mental meanderings can lead to a spiral of overeating, self-loathing, depression and insomnia. Saying 'Pull yourself together' rarely works. But you *can* counter these negative thoughts by practising mindful meditation. Instead of obsessing, you can take time out to look at yourself and your thoughts in a less judgmental, more reasonable way.

Mindful meditation, also known as 'mindfulness', is a modern take on the ancient practice of meditation. The good news is you don't need to be religious or go on a retreat to a Tibetan monastery to do it. What you are trying to do is spend a short amount of time every day focusing your awareness on the present moment, rather than worrying about the past or making plans for the future. You don't try to ignore thoughts and feelings, which inevitably intrude; you just notice and accept them, without engaging with them. I find it useful to think of negative thoughts and feelings as being like leaves falling into a stream, which you notice but which are soon gone.

Mindful meditation was developed by a cognitive scientist called Jon Kabat-Zinn in the 1970s. He was interested in using Buddhist-inspired practices to reduce stress and studying the benefits through scientific research. Since the 1970s there have been more than 8000 studies involving mindful meditation.

The clinically proven benefits really are both widespread and impressive.

Brain scans have shown mindfulness can increase the density of grey matter in areas of the brain involved in regulating emotion, learning and memory. Just six weeks of daily practice are enough to trigger measurable improvements in insomnia, fatigue and depression and reductions in anxiety and stress. This impact on stress has even been found to help regulate blood sugar levels.

Dr Sara Lazar is an associate professor in psychology at Harvard Medical School and a specialist in the neuroscience of meditation. Her studies have shown that regular mindfulness can change the areas of the brain associated with fear and other strong emotions.

'We have seen the amygdala – the main "fight or flight" area of the brain – get smaller,' she told me. 'The smaller it becomes, the less stress people report. Although exercise is good for reducing stress, it can't change the shape of the amygdala in the same way.'

Her studies show regular mindfulness can decrease pain perception and improve memory. 'We found regular mindfulness can trigger positive changes to the hippocampus – the part of the brain which handles memory and attention. This part naturally declines with age, but mindfulness appears to give it a boost,' she says.

In Dr Lazar's studies, the volunteers practised every day for 40 minutes over eight weeks, but she says there are great benefits to be had from practising 10–15 minutes a day several times a week.

The more you do it, the easier it gets, and ultimately you should be able to switch on the calming benefits of mindfulness mode whenever you need it (which is usually when your mind is at its most active).

Try this simple exercise.

MINDFUL BREATHING

Set aside time every day to do this. It doesn't have to be in the morning; some people prefer the afternoon or evening – do whatever suits you.

Sit in a comfortable chair, in a room where you won't be disturbed. Rest your hands on your thighs, soften your focus, or close your eyes, then for the next few minutes try to focus on your breath.

Notice the way the air goes through your nose or mouth, and the way that your belly rises and falls. If you find it helps, count your breaths going in and out, in units of 10.

Notice the weight of your hands on your thighs, and the feeling of your feet on the floor. When your thoughts drift back to the cares of the day, which they will, try to gently bring your focus back to your breathing.

I imagine my mind as a wild horse that resents being restrained in this way. To start with, you will find the horse constantly wants to bolt. Just bring it gently back to the breath and the present moment. Over time the horse will get used to it.

You may find this easier to do, certainly to start with, if you join a group or download a mindfulness app, like Calm or Headspace. If you do it with an app they will probably recommend you start with just a couple of minutes at a time, before building up to 10 minutes or more.

Both my sister, Susie Stead, and my brother-in-law, Tim Stead, teach mindfulness at the world-renowned Oxford Mindfulness Centre. These are a couple of their suggestions for other ways of building mindfulness into your day:

MINDFUL MOMENTS

When you get up in the morning, set your mobile phone alarm for some random time in the day. When it goes off, stop what you are doing and look around. Notice where you are, who else is around and what thoughts were going through your mind when the alarm went off. Ask yourself what your mood is like. How are you feeling? Check in with your body. How's that knee? Have a think about what you would like to do next – not what you always do, perhaps something different. The point of this exercise is to shake up your normal routine and make you realise you have choices.

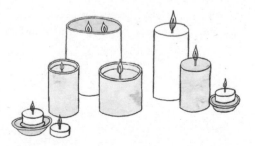

MINDFULNESS IN NATURE

Go outside, to a nearby park, wood or field. Find an interesting tree or some flowers and look at them. Really look at them. You don't need to know their name; just spend time admiring their colours, their patterns, the way they grow. As you do this, your mind will wander. You will start thinking about what you need to do next or what you are going to have for your next meal. Try coming back to the flower. Just for a few minutes.

NOTE: Mindfulness can cause old memories to unexpectedly resurface, so if you have a history of trauma seek the guidance of a good mental health professional.

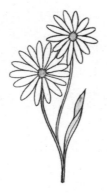

The more you do it,
the easier it gets,
and ultimately you
should be able to
switch on the calming
benefits of mindfulness
mode whenever you
need it (which is usually
when your mind is at
its most active).

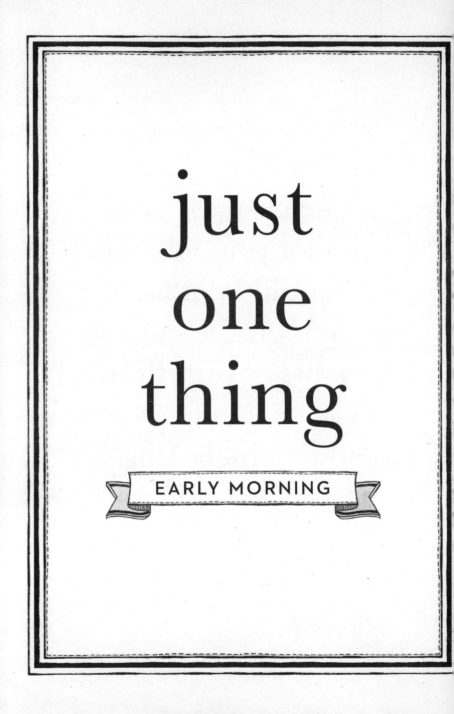

just one thing

EARLY MORNING

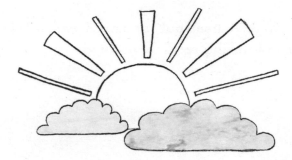

early-morning walk

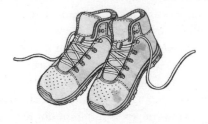

How to do it: head out for a brisk walk within two hours of waking up each morning.

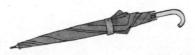

I've saved the best Just One Thing for last in this section – taking an early-morning walk. This is something that I swear by – it is surprisingly life-changing. Believe it or not, getting out and about first thing – within an hour or two of getting up – can improve your sleep, boost your mood, increase your fitness and cut your risk of heart disease and diabetes.

I love morning walks. Even when it is cold and wet, I still set off with boots and a brolly. Heading out early (ideally within two hours of waking up) means you get the health benefits not only of the exercise, but also of exposure to natural light. And if you go for your walk in a green space, like a wood or a park, even better. Best of all, take a dog. Both of you will really appreciate it.

The first thing that I notice, when I step outside with our dog, Tari, excitedly yapping at my heels, is just how bright it is. Light levels outdoors are at least 10 times brighter than inside your house, and when this light hits sensors at the back of your eyes, this sends messages to a part of your brain called the pituitary gland, ordering it to stop producing the hormone melatonin. Melatonin is known as 'the hormone of darkness' because rising levels, in the evening, help put you to sleep at night.

As well as waking you up, bright outdoor light helps reset your internal body clock, which in turn helps to regulate hunger, mood, body temperature and all sorts of other important bodily processes. This resetting of the internal clock also means that at the other end of the day, when you head for bed, you are ready to sleep.

Research shows that the earlier your exposure to bright light, the greater the impact on your quality, and quantity, of sleep. In a study carried out in 2017, office workers were asked to wear light-measuring devices for one week in summer, and then again in winter. They also kept a record of their sleep and filled in questionnaires about their mood.

The researchers found that people who were exposed to the most light during the morning hours fell asleep faster and had fewer sleep disturbances during the night. They were also less likely to report feelings of depression and stress.

A short morning walk can be a great way to boost your mood if, like me and many other people, you suffer from seasonal affective disorder (SAD), also known as the winter blues. During the long winter months, we tend to spend more time indoors and are therefore exposed to far less daylight, which can throw our circadian rhythms out of sync. Exposure to bright daylight also triggers the release of a neurotransmitter called serotonin, a natural mood-booster that is lower in people with SAD.

Ideally, you need to be outside for 30 minutes to get the full benefits. If you don't have the time for that long a walk, or you live somewhere that has dark and gloomy mornings, you could invest in a SAD lamp, a screen that produces at least 10,000 lux of light (typical indoor lighting is more like 200 lux). I use mine in winter and prop it up beside me while I am having breakfast or working on the computer.

If you can, however, do try and fit in a morning walk. As well as exposing you to lots of light, any walk – short, long, fast or slow –

will strengthen muscles and bones, reduce joint and muscular pain, burn a few calories and increase energy levels.

And if you want to supercharge your daily walk, just speed it up to the sort of pace you'd use if you were in a hurry to get somewhere. A brisk walk means aiming to be doing around 100 paces a minute, which you will find easier to achieve if you listen to music with a suitable beat (see box opposite). You could even fit in another Just One Thing by singing along to it.

Not only does brisk walking increase your fitness, compared to a more leisurely dawdle, it might even extend your life. A 2018 study by the University of Ulster looked at the walking habits of 50,000 people and found that those who regularly went on brisk walks were 24 per cent less likely to die over the time period being studied compared to those who reported walking slowly.

Brisk walking increases your heart rate, placing a greater demand on your cardiovascular system, thereby maintaining cardio fitness and helping to lower blood pressure. Which is why brisk walkers have a 21 per cent lower risk of death from heart disease than their more sedentary friends.

If a 30-minute walk is unrealistic, try dividing your walking time into three 10-minute chunks. This will not only break up the time you spend sitting, but also give your metabolism a mini-boost, keeping it elevated throughout the day.

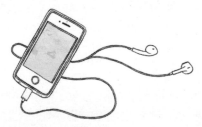

GET WITH THE BEAT

A brisk walk means doing around 100 paces, or 'beats', per minute. If you have a music-streaming service you can search for 100bpm tracks to create your own walking playlist, but try these popular classics for starters:

Beyoncé – Crazy in Love
Shakira – Hips Don't Lie
Lynyrd Skynyrd – Sweet Home Alabama
KT Tunstall – Suddenly I See
Maroon 5 – She Will Be Loved
Stevie Wonder – Superstition
ABBA – Dancing Queen
Imagine Dragons – On Top of the World
U2 – I Still Haven't Found What I'm Looking For
Prince – Let's Go Crazy
Tears for Fears – Shout
Wilson Phillips – Hold On

BEFORE OR AFTER BREAKFAST?

To be honest, this is very much down to what works for you. If you eat breakfast, then a brisk walk afterwards will help burn off some of the sugar and fat that would otherwise be running round your system. On the other hand, a fasting walk (i.e. walking on an empty stomach) could help nudge you into fat-burning mode.

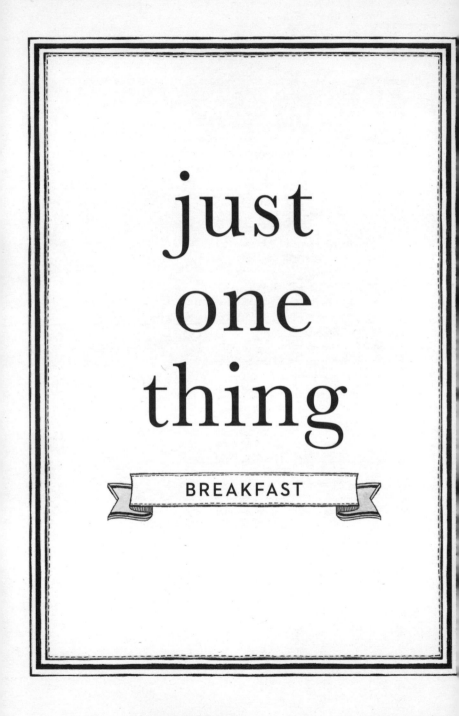

just one thing

BREAKFAST

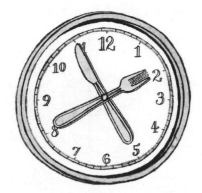

change your mealtimes

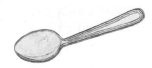

How to do it: delay your breakfast by an hour and try not to eat within three hours of going to bed.

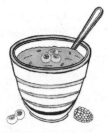

When you get up in the morning, you may well be in a rush and keen to tuck into your breakfast and get out of the door. Or you may be perfectly happy to hold off eating for a while (a lot of people find they don't get hungry until later in the day).

One reason why you might want to delay having breakfast if you're not ravenous is that, by doing so, you will be extending your overnight fast (i.e. how long it has been since your last meal).

Extending your overnight fast is known as time-restricted eating (TRE), and is based on research showing the multiple health benefits to be had from having a slightly later breakfast and an earlier evening meal (and, of course, no late-night snack!). TRE is a very popular form of intermittent fasting and is sometimes also known as 16:8 or 14:10.

16:8 is the more challenging version of TRE, involving fasting for 16 hours, and only eating within an eight-hour window. It may be more effective to do this, but it is tougher to stick to. Personally, I think that anyone who manages an overnight fast of more than 12 hours is doing well, particularly as many of us have got into the habit of eating from soon after we wake up until last thing at night, when we have a snack or a milky drink.

The idea of restricting the hours within which you eat is hardly new. More than 2000 years ago, the Buddha advocated not eating after midday, because he said the practice put him in 'good health'. Now modern science suggests the Buddha could have been on to something.

I first came across the science of TRE in 2012 when I was writing a book called *The Fast Diet*, all about different forms of fasting and calorie restriction. As I explained in the introduction, the book focused on a novel approach that I was testing, which I called 5:2 (where you cut your food intake two days a week and eat normally on the other five), but I also looked into the science behind TRE. At the time, the most prominent scientist working on TRE was Professor Satchin Panda of the Salk Institute in California. He had recently published a study where they took two groups of mice and fed them a high-fat diet. Both groups of mice got the same amount of food, but one group were allowed to eat it whenever they wanted, while the other group had to eat all their food in an eight-hour period.

After 100 days, there were some dramatic differences between the two groups. The mice who had eaten whenever they wanted now had much higher levels of cholesterol and blood sugars, and had put on far more weight (28 per cent more) than the mice who had to fast for 16 hours a day.

Since then, there have been numerous studies in humans showing that extending your overnight fast and eating within a shortened daytime window can lower your blood pressure and cholesterol levels, help you lose weight, improve your sleep, cut your risk of developing type 2 diabetes, and may even slow the rate at which the brain declines as we age.

As Professor Panda showed, a lot of this is down to our internal body clocks which control our circadian rhythm – the natural process which regulates our sleep–wake cycle. Eating late at night, when the body is preparing for sleep, can throw our body out of sync. It also means that the fat and sugar we've just consumed will hang around in our bloodstream for far longer than it would if it had been eaten earlier in the day, which is bad news for our heart and has the potential to disrupt our sleep.

Professor Panda told me that he personally follows a 14:10 approach, and this is also where a lot of modern research is focused. His preferred eating pattern is to have breakfast around 8am (roughly two hours after he wakes up) and then have an evening meal with his family around 6pm, which gives him 14 hours of overnight fasting.

I recently interviewed another leading researcher from the Salk Institute, Dr Emily Manoogian, who is also a specialist in body clocks and circadian rhythms. '*What* you eat and *how much* you eat is always going to be important, but we now know that *when* you eat is an important third component of good nutrition,' she told me.

Dr Manoogian agrees that eating at all hours of the day and night, as so many of us do, disrupts the body's natural circadian rhythm, which really wants most systems to be more active during the day and dormant at night.

'Sleep is when your body should be in a state of rest and repair, but if you go to bed having eaten throughout the evening, your body will have to focus on digestion instead,' she says. 'You can end up with elevated blood glucose levels all night, which increases your risk of diabetes.

'Chronic disruption to this system leads to increased rates of disease and weight gain, blood pressure and inflammation.

But by restricting the time window in which we eat we can powerfully support our circadian system, and this can go a long way to help our bodies function better.'

As a bonus, TRE can lead to modest weight loss – mainly because you are cutting out the late-night snacking. And, because your body isn't having to digest lots of food late at night, it can also improve your sleep. In fact, Dr Manoogian's studies have found that when you stop eating three to four hours before bed, you sleep better and wake up feeling more rested the next day.

She recommends incorporating TRE as part of a healthy lifestyle, regardless of your current state of health, and suggests choosing an 8–10 hour eating window that works best for you, one you can happily stick to every single day of the week.

Ideally, she says, start your window one or two hours after you wake up in the morning, and end it three to four hours before you go to bed. 'If possible, aim to eat most of your calories in the first half of your day, and for best results, aim to have a consistent eight hours in bed each night,' she adds.

Outside of the eating window, while you are effectively 'fasting', she recommends drinking only water – hot or cold. 'Milk is a hard no,' she says. 'Some clinical trials accept black tea and coffee but there is a debate about how caffeine affects glucose regulation, so stick to hot or cold water outside of your eating window if you can.'

I asked Steph to give it a go.

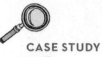

CASE STUDY
Steff

'Breakfast for me has always been at 8am, and I used to graze through the day, snacking on biscuits in front of the TV until about 10.30 at night. But extending my nine hours of 'fasting' to 14 hours means I have to skip breakfast and say no to those late-night snacks. I confess, the toughest challenge has been stopping eating at 7pm. It helps that I can still eat chocolate during my eating hours, but I have to admit I do cheat occasionally. The biggest change is shifting my main meal to 2pm each day – it works really well, and it means I'm no longer starving hungry and looking for snacks when I get home from work at 5pm.'

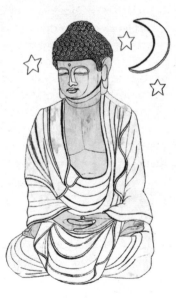

More than 2000 years ago the Buddha advocated not eating after midday, because he said the practice put him in 'good health'. Now modern science suggests the Buddha could have been on to something.

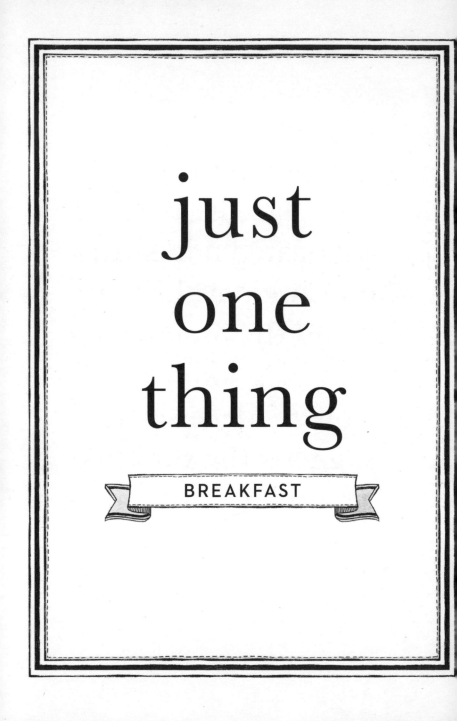

just one thing

BREAKFAST

drink
water

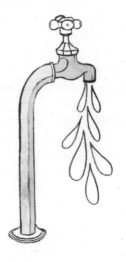

How to do it: try to drink a glass of water with every meal.

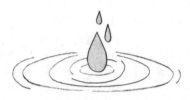

For many of us a cup of coffee or tea is something we grab almost as soon as we wake. There's no doubt both are reviving, but it may be best to wait till you are having breakfast for a major caffeine fix (see page 76). Instead, why not try knocking back a large glass of water? Studies show that keeping adequately hydrated can improve attention and help with problem solving; it also enhances physical performance, helps you keep calm and can boost your mood.

Water makes up 60 per cent of our bodies and 90 per cent of our brains, so it is not surprising that it plays a central part in our lives. We need water to hydrate our skin, digest food and enable our kidneys to flush out waste. It's also very important to replace the water we lose in sweat, especially if it's hot or if we're exercising.

Water is so critical to our brains that even losing 1–2 per cent of it is enough to impair our cognitive function. That's why rehydration studies have shown that drinking more water leads to improvements in both working and short-term memory, and can significantly reduce regular headaches.

Drinking more water could also help you lose weight. In a recent study, two groups adopted the same weight loss diet, but one group were asked to drink a pint of water before each meal. That group ended up consuming fewer calories and lost the most weight.

So how do you judge when and how much to drink? Some people suggest that thirst is the most obvious clue, but as Stuart Galloway, professor of exercise physiology at the University of Stirling, told me, we shouldn't wait until we feel thirsty.

'By the time you notice thirst, your fluid content is probably down by 1–2 per cent of your body mass, which is quite low,' he says. 'At this level, dehydration can affect your physical abilities and also some of your mental faculties, as well as your mood, and induce a feeling of fatigue.'

Professor Galloway recommends sticking to the European guidelines of drinking around two litres a day for men and 1.6 litres for women: 'Use urine colour (it should be pale yellow) and the number of times you go to the loo as a guide,' he adds. 'Aim to be making six or seven trips to the lavatory a day – if you only go three or four times, you're probably not drinking enough.'

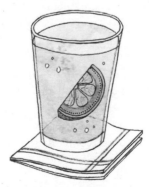

So, along with your '5 a day' (the amount of fruit and veg you should eat each day), here is another number to remember: '7 a day': the number of trips to make to the loo in a 24-hour period.

'You can have tea and coffee as part of your liquid intake, but once you start on your fifth cup of coffee the caffeine might start to have a diuretic effect,' he warns.

Drinking a glass of water with each meal will help you meet your daily fluid intake targets and will ensure you remain hydrated throughout the day. I think water is great. It contains no calories, it's free and it's delicious (particularly if you drink it chilled, with a slice of lemon).

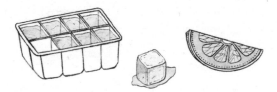

Drinking more water could even help you lose weight. In a recent study, two groups adopted the same weight loss diet, but one group were asked to drink a pint of water before each meal. That group ended up consuming fewer calories and lost the most weight.

just one thing

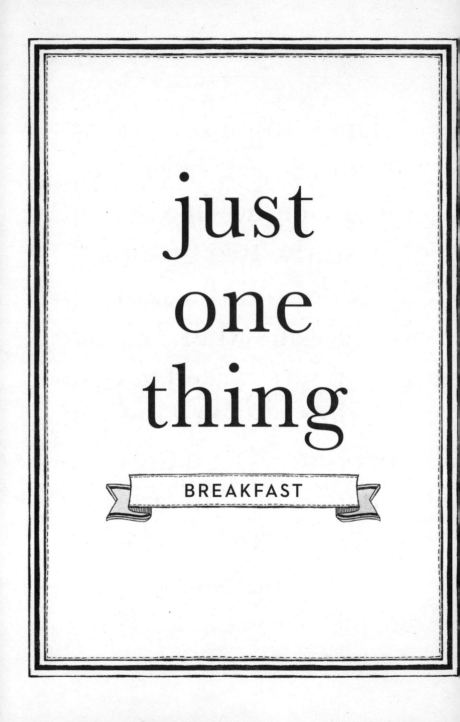

BREAKFAST

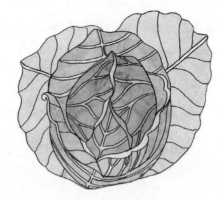

eat some
bacteria

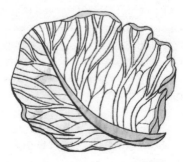

How to do it: try eating sauerkraut or other fermented foods, like kimchi or kefir.

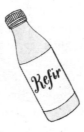

Whether or not you decide to delay your breakfast (and some people skip it altogether), the big question is: what are you going to eat? In Victorian times, the middle classes ate fish, eggs and meat for breakfast, while the poor ate porridge or gruel. Then, in 1894, Dr John Harvey Kellogg and his brother, William Keith, began to make and promote cornflakes (flakes of maize which were later flavoured with sugar) as a healthy start to the day.

Dr Kellogg, a prominent eugenicist who advocated sterilising 'mentally defective persons', also believed that eating cornflakes would drain the sexual energy of young people and stop them masturbating, a terrible activity which he claimed caused cancer of the womb, urinary diseases, impotence, epilepsy, insanity and even death. 'Such a victim', he wrote, 'literally dies by his own hand.'

I'm not a big fan of breakfast cereals, as many of them can be up to 35 per cent sugar. I prefer kippers, porridge with toasted walnuts or eggs for breakfast. Eggs are a great source of protein and will keep you fuller for longer. And with my eggs I often eat a big dollop of homemade purple sauerkraut.

I find the tangy pickled cabbage really brings out the creamy taste of the eggs, but I also enjoy eating it because it is bursting with beneficial bacteria.

Fermentation is an excellent food preservation method that has been used for thousands of years. More lately, fermented foods have become super trendy because of multiple claims about their health benefits, such as weight loss and stronger immunity, only some of which have been scientifically tested.

One thing that's certain is that in recent years there has been a surge of research into the gut microbiome – the thousands of different species of microbes living in your gut that have a profound effect on your health. The gut microbiome is made up of around a hundred trillion microbes – a mixture of bacteria, viruses and fungi. Together they weigh up to 2kg – more than your brain. They make up about half the cells in your body, which means, if you think about it, you are half human and half microbiome.

Indeed, a scientist once estimated that, because faeces are largely made up of bacteria, every time you empty your bowels you become – briefly – slightly more human than microbe.

Your gut microbiome is like a complex rainforest; and, like a rainforest, it hosts a rich diversity of life, all battling for survival. Some of these gut microbes seem to be good for our health; others less so.

We know the microbiome can influence our immune system and alter the activity of things like our natural killer cells, a vital part of our body's defences. Some of them are very adept at turning the fibre in our diet into anti-inflammatory compounds, which are hugely beneficial because chronic inflammation leads to conditions like type 2 diabetes, heart disease and dementia.

But perhaps the most surprising discovery is the link between the gut and the brain. There are certain gut microbes, it seems, that have an impact on our mood. There's even a new word to describe these microbes: psychobiotics.

Dr Kirsten Berding Harold is a dietitian and microbiome specialist from University College Cork. She told me that it is probably the anti-inflammatory powers of these microbes that have the positive effect on mental health.

One of her most recent studies showed that switching volunteers to a diet packed with wholegrains and vegetables plus two to three servings of kefir (a zingy form of fermented milk), sauerkraut or kimchi (a Korean take on sauerkraut) each day resulted in noticeably lowered stress levels and improved mood scores in just four weeks.

Dr Berding Harold and her team are currently exploring the use of a gut-friendly diet as a supplementary therapy for people with treatment-resistant depression.

But don't expect instant miracles with your first spoonful of sauerkraut. Dr Berding Harold recommends adopting a wholefood diet and avoiding foods that can have a toxic effect on gut bacteria (i.e. processed foods full of fat, salt and sugar), and then layering the fermented foods on top. Incidentally, introducing fermented foods to your diet can result in a lot of gas, so do start slowly!

HOW TO BOOST YOUR GOOD BACTERIA

You can buy sauerkraut, kombucha (fermented tea) and kefir in large supermarkets – but do check they contain live bacteria. Personally, I think it is better, and much cheaper, if you make it yourself.

Dr Clare Bailey's purple sauerkraut
200g beetroot (grated)
1kg red cabbage (finely sliced)
½ small apple, peeled, cored and finely chopped
1 tsp fennel seeds
1 tsp coriander seeds
2 tbsp crystal sea salt
Large 1 litre glass jar with a secure lid

Make sure you wash your hands thoroughly. Then, wearing rubber gloves to avoid staining your hands, mix all the ingredients together in a large bowl and massage vigorously to soften the cabbage until the salt draws out fluid. Then cram the mixture, including the juices, into a clean, re-sealable glass jar, leaving about 2cm space at the top for the mixture to bubble and fizz. The veg should sit below the level of the juices (you may need to add filtered water to make sure it does). Close the lid and leave the jar at room temperature, opening it daily and pressing the veg down to release the bubbles for about a week. Taste it occasionally. If it is not ready, keep going for 10 days or so (the longer you leave it, the more sour it becomes). When ready, your sauerkraut can be kept in the fridge for several months. It should smell sweet and tangy.

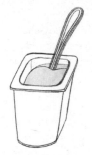

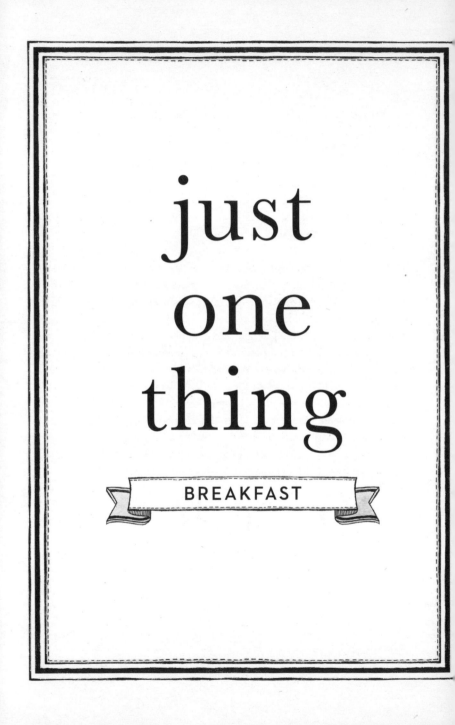

just one thing

BREAKFAST

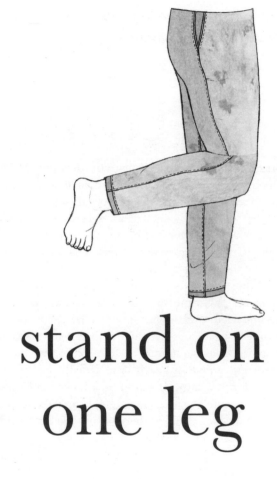

stand on
one leg

How to do it: raise one leg and use your core muscles to help you balance.

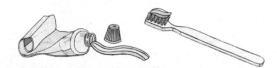

After breakfast it is, of course, time to brush your teeth. And, if you were to pop your head around the bathroom door when I'm brushing mine, you'd see me standing on one leg. I do it for two minutes, switching legs every 30 seconds or so. Sometimes, if I'm feeling brave, I even close my eyes and focus hard on trying not to wobble.

I do this to improve my balance, and the reason for this is research that shows that by improving my balance, I am reducing my risk of injury, improving my posture and possibly even adding years to my life. Falls, it turns out, are the second-commonest cause of accidental deaths, worldwide, after traffic accidents. And having a good sense of balance is critical to reducing the risk of a fall.

Balance is something most of us take for granted but it's like muscle strength – use it or lose it! And actually standing upright, on two legs, is pretty hard. It wasn't till around 6 million years ago that our remote ancestors managed to do it consistently, a development which enabled them to spot predators and free their hands to make tools.

When you are standing upright, the main things that are keeping you from falling over are messages from sensors in your inner ear, muscles, joints and eyes. They work together to tell your brain where your body is in space, allowing you to unconsciously shift your weight so you don't tumble.

We start to lose our ability to balance – like so many other things – when we enter our forties and fifties, and we don't really think about it until we topple or fall.

Indeed, there is some evidence that our modern sedentary lifestyle is causing our ability to balance to decline more rapidly than in previous generations. I was told by Dawn Skelton, an exercise physiologist and professor of ageing and health at Glasgow Caledonian University, that 'good balance requires you to be on your feet regularly, and with each generation we have become progressively less active, spending more time sitting behind screens'.

But the good news is that studies show that you can, swiftly, improve your balance. This will have a positive effect on your core strength and your co-ordination. And because balance involves a remarkable feat of co-ordination between your muscles, inner ear and eyes, it is also a great predictor of how well you are ageing.

In a study which started back in 1999, researchers from the UK's Medical Research Council did three simple tests on 2760 men and women who, at that time, were all 53 years old. The tests included measuring their grip strength, how quickly they could stand upright from sitting and how long they could stand on one leg with their eyes closed.

When the researchers returned 13 years later, they discovered that 177 of the volunteers had died: 88 from cancer, 47 from heart disease, and 42 from other causes. And when they combed through their data, they found that the test that had *best* predicted the chance that someone would die was the one-legged eyes-closed test. Those who did poorly – who could only manage a couple of seconds – were three times more likely to have died than those who could stay standing for 10 seconds or more.

So why is balance such a good predictor of healthy ageing? I asked Professor Skelton. 'Good balance requires your brain to integrate information from lots of places around the body, and any problems could be a sign that your body is struggling to integrate and act on all that information,' she told me.

'If your brain isn't doing well for balance, it might not be doing so well in the co-ordination of other important areas such as hormones and cardiovascular systems,' she added.

If you want to try this test, you will need to get a friend with a watch or mobile phone with a stopwatch. Start by taking off your shoes. Now put your hands on your hips and stand on one leg. When you are ready, close your eyes. You will be dismayed how quickly you start to sway. The test is over as soon as you shift your planted foot or when you have to put your raised foot down on the ground to stop yourself falling. To get an accurate score, take an average of three attempts.

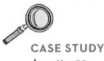

CASE STUDY

Annette, 50

'When I tried the one-legged 'tree' balance during a yoga class, I made a very wobbly tree, so I was keen to see if regular daily practice would help. At first I could only stand on one leg for a few seconds. But I was quickly able to extend the amount of time I could manage. It is certainly easier if you keep your eyes open and focused on a point on the wall. When I closed my eyes, though, I really noticed how my core muscles were forced into action. It is definitely getting easier and I'm confident I'll be a yoga tree professional in no time!'

HOW LONG SHOULD YOU BE ABLE TO BALANCE ON ONE LEG?

The following numbers are based on a study in which American researchers asked people from different age groups to balance on one leg so they could tell what 'normal' looks like.

People under 40 with eyes open averaged 45 seconds.
With eyes closed: 15 seconds.
People aged 40-49 with eyes open averaged 42 seconds.
With eyes closed: 13 seconds.
People aged 50-59 with eyes open averaged 41 seconds.
With eyes closed: 8 seconds.
People aged 60-69 with eyes open averaged 32 seconds.
With eyes closed: 4 seconds.
People aged 70-79 with eyes open averaged 22 seconds.
With eyes closed: 3 seconds.

To improve your balance you could try yoga, tai chi, using a 'wobble board', walking backwards (be careful) or just standing on one leg when you brush your teeth or boil the kettle – as I do. If you can integrate balance exercises into your everyday routine, it really could have a life-changing impact. Fewer falls means less chance of fractures. You'll be boosting your core strength, posture and co-ordination. You are also more likely to walk upright rather than hunched, which will make you look younger and might even improve your mood.

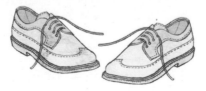

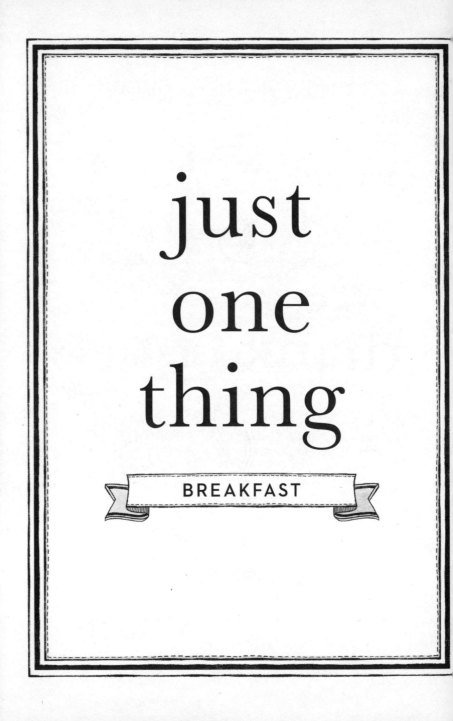

just one thing

BREAKFAST

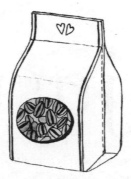

drink coffee

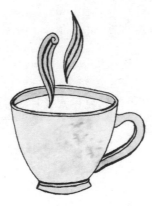

How to do it: drink one to three cups of coffee a day.

For many of you, having a lovely cup of coffee is probably Just One Thing that is already deeply ingrained in your daily routine. However, those of you who drink it first thing in the morning might want to think about delaying your first cup a little, and here's why.

Firstly, you are better off drinking coffee *after* brushing your teeth, rather than before. (I wouldn't recommend drinking it straight away – the taste might be a bit peculiar. Wait until your mouth has had time to remove those toothpaste flavours.) Drinking your coffee after brushing means you are less likely to damage and stain your teeth. This is because coffee is acidic and can weaken your enamel, the outer, protective layer of your teeth. If you brush your teeth immediately after drinking, it is like applying sandpaper; it causes micro-abrasions. It is also more likely to stain your teeth because, although coffee doesn't stain enamel, it does stain plaque, which hopefully you will have removed with assiduous flossing and brushing.

Another reason for delaying your coffee until after brushing your teeth is that pouring coffee down your throat first thing in the morning is not great for your body. Or at least that is what Dr James Betts, who is professor of metabolic physiology at the University of Bath, told me.

'For most of us', he said, 'our remedy for a bad night's sleep is to wake up and have a nice strong coffee. But this is a bad thing for your body because poor sleep raises levels of the stress hormone, cortisol, which can then push your blood sugar levels up to unhealthy highs.'

It turns out that drinking coffee first thing compounds both these issues. Indeed, Professor Betts has done studies that show that drinking coffee straight after a poor night's sleep can lead to a 50 per cent bigger surge in your blood sugar levels when you have breakfast than if you delay the coffee until after eating.

Even if you have slept well, you will still experience a rise in your cortisol levels (this is known as CAR, or cortisol arousal response), which starts a couple of hours before you wake and peaks an hour or so after you get up.

So it is best to hit your body with caffeine when your cortisol levels are falling, not while they are still high. If you drink coffee when cortisol levels are high, you will soon develop tolerance to it; in other words, you will find you need to drink more of it to get the same kick.

For both these reasons Professor Betts recommends delaying that first coffee until breakfast or later to minimise its negative effects on your blood sugar levels.

So why drink coffee at all? As well as the fact that I love the taste and it perks me up, it provides lots of health benefits. Coffee is rich in flavanols and antioxidants called polyphenols – compounds shown to promote better brain and heart health, and to have anti-inflammatory effects. Studies suggest that coffee drinkers have lower rates of stroke, heart disease, cancer and dementia.

In fact, a single dose of caffeine is enough to enhance attention, alertness, contentment and mood.

Coffee aficionados will also be delighted to hear that their favourite brew may even help burn calories. A Nottingham University study showed that drinking a coffee stimulates the activity of brown fat, which helps to generate body heat by burning calories. This claim is supported by recent research showing that women who drank two or three cups of coffee a day had less total body fat, and abdominal fat, than those who didn't drink any.

But the thing that surprises me most is the impact of coffee and caffeine on athletic performance and endurance. According to Professor Betts, caffeine is one of the most effective supplements an athlete can take: 'It is very clear that the effects of caffeine are not only large, but really wide-ranging across almost every aspect of performance, whether it's our cognitive ability, strength, explosive speed, endurance or skill. All of these things can benefit from caffeine and coffee. Despite the number of supplements athletes take, I genuinely feel you can count on one hand the things that actually work. And I put caffeine at the top of that list, both for the size of effect that you get and the breadth.'

To get the most out of it, you should drink coffee about an hour before exercising, because it takes that long to peak in your system. Similarly, if you are driving late at night and feeling sleepy, your best bet is to stop at a service station, drink a cup of coffee, go back to your car for a 30–40-minute snooze, then drive on.

So how much coffee should you drink? The optimal dose seems to be around three cups a day – and no more than five. Your ability to metabolise caffeine (clear it out of your system) and your sensitivity to it depend largely on your personal genetics. I'm sensitive to caffeine, but I am also a fast metaboliser, meaning I clear it from my system very quickly. I've discovered that my blood pressure shoots up after I drink coffee (which is one of the unfortunate side effects of drinking the stuff), but it also falls again within a couple of hours.

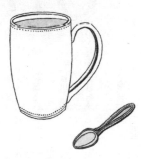

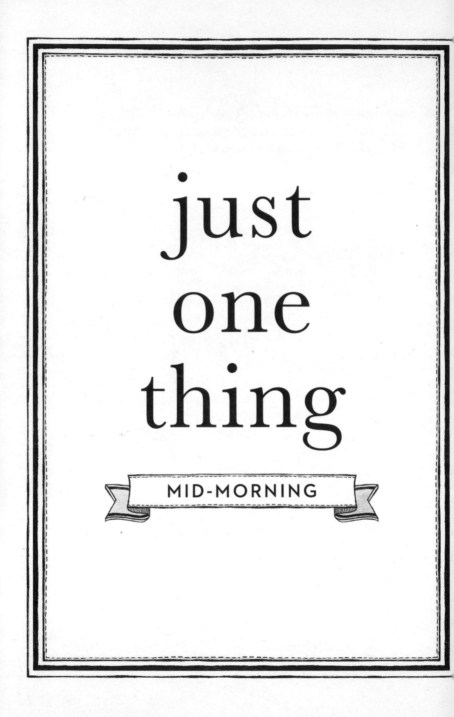

just one thing

MID-MORNING

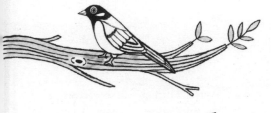

take a
break

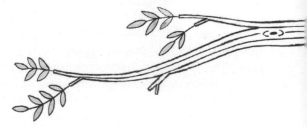

How to do it: down tools and take a break a few times a day.

These days, as well as making TV programmes (and podcasts), I spend a lot of time writing. And it never gets any easier. I am a great procrastinator and I find any excuse not to sit down and start. I need the fear of a deadline to get me going, but when I finally begin, I quickly become totally immersed in what I am doing and loathe to break off in case I get distracted. Research shows, however, that I could be much more productive and creative if I moved away from my desk and spent a few minutes wandering around the garden at intervals throughout the day.

It turns out that, far from being self-indulgent, taking a break, particularly if you get up and move around, could make you more engaged and more productive, and enhance your enjoyment of work. It can also have a big impact on psychological stress. Studies have shown that micro-breaks can lower levels of the stress hormone cortisol, making you more effective in the long run. And, if, like me, you tend to hunch over your desk or slump in front of the TV, regular mini-breaks which require you to stand up or walk about are a golden opportunity to improve your posture and ease joint pain.

The idea that we might all benefit from micro-breaks emerged from research carried out in the late 1980s in the US. The researchers found that the workers who took slightly longer breaks – up to about three minutes – not only produced more accurate work, but had lower heart rates, suggesting that taking the breaks had a calming effect.

Since then, more evidence has stacked up showing that taking short breaks seems to have a disproportionately powerful effect on how well you work.

In a fascinating study in which surgeons, performing complex laparoscopic surgery, were randomly allocated to either taking a five-minute break every 30 minutes or no breaks at all, researchers found those who got the breaks made fewer mistakes than those who just had to power through. AND, surprisingly, taking a break didn't make the operations any longer.

Another study involving surgeons found that taking micro-breaks improved accuracy and reduced levels of fatigue by half.

Although it is best if you get up and wander around, doing something as simple as regularly looking away from your screen could improve your eye health. Just follow the 20-20-20 rule: look away from your screen every 20 minutes for 20 seconds, focusing on an object 20 feet away. Try it – it works!

And don't feel guilty if you, like many of us, drift off into daydreaming! Neuroscientist Professor Moshe Bar at Bar-Ilan University in Tel Aviv has just written a book on 'mind wandering' and he told me that breaking off to occasionally let your mind wander will boost creativity. 'Mind wandering is a power tool for creative thinking,' he says. 'It helps to improve mood, decision making and mental resilience.' He believes we should all break off from whatever we are doing and allocate some time to daydreaming every day.

'Creative thinking requires a stage called "incubation",' he says. 'The decision-making process starts with "divergent thinking", where you create as many ideas as possible; then you need a period of incubation to allow your subconscious brain to evaluate all these ideas, before you can move into "convergent thinking", which fine-tunes the process to the best single solution. This process requires downtime so you can incubate all your thoughts.'

I love this! Next time a publisher or editor chases me for work I might tell them it's 'incubating'!

Professor Bar warns that taking a break won't be anywhere near as effective if you spend it watching TV or scrolling through your social media channels: 'To give your brain the best chance to wander creatively you shouldn't load it with anything else,' he says, 'but you can optimise the break by nudging your thoughts in the direction of positive subjects rather than allowing yourself to worry about unpaid bills.'

All you have to do is break off from what you are doing every so often, look away and let your mind go – what could be simpler?

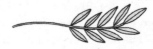

Neuroscientist Professor Moshe Bar at Bar-Ilan University in Tel Aviv believes we should all break off from whatever we are doing and allocate some time to daydreaming every day.

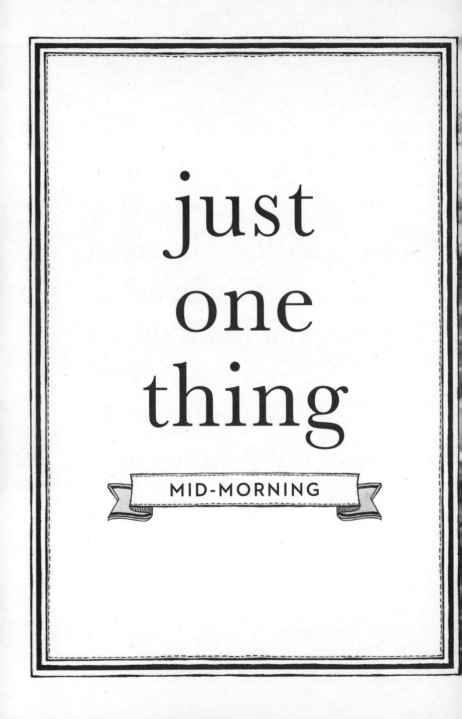

just one thing

MID-MORNING

deep breaths

How to do it: spend a few minutes each day practising slow, controlled breathing.

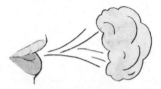

This is one of my favourite Just One Things. It's a perfect example of something that is simple, quick and completely life-changing; it can transform your mood and your health, and bring a quiet joy to your day.

That's because just by changing how quickly and deeply you breathe, you can achieve amazing things: you can slow your heart rate, lower your blood pressure, reduce stress levels and combat anxiety. There is also evidence that changing the way you breathe can reduce pain.

That said, taking slow, deep breaths is surprisingly difficult, particularly when you are stressed, so it pays to practise every day. That way it becomes an automatic 'go to' response when you need it most.

'Slow breathing is an incredibly potent way of giving yourself a mini-tranquiliser,' says Ian Robertson, who is emeritus professor of psychology at Trinity College Dublin and one of the leading experts in the science of wellbeing, 'and yet a lot of the time we forget to do it.'

'When very busy or stressed we tend to hold our breath, or breathe more rapidly, which can make us feel more panicked; and unless we have made deep breathing a very well-practised habit, we are unlikely to do it in time to glean its benefits,' he says.

'You can calm things down by slowing your breathing, and you will be surprised at how quickly you feel better, but it is hard to get into the habit of doing it, particularly if you're feeling stressed. So I just try to remember to take slow breaths in for a count of four and out for a count of six whenever I pause or change activity.'

So how does slow breathing work? Professor Robertson told me that, among other things, there are special sensors in the brain that detect carbon dioxide levels in the blood and rapidly respond by either releasing, or inhibiting the release of, a chemical messenger called noradrenaline. This is the brain's equivalent of adrenaline for the body, and it triggers the 'fight or flight' response, which can get us out of trouble, or equally, cause us to feel stressed and anxious.

'When you slow your breathing, you change carbon dioxide levels in your blood, and this reduces the levels of noradrenaline, which helps make you feel calm,' he says. 'Slow breathing also triggers the parasympathetic autonomic nervous system, which causes your heart to slow and your blood pressure to drop, and this has an additional calming effect.'

Many studies show that controlling your breathing can be a really effective way to control anxiety. And performing breathing exercises can also improve your decision making because, as Professor Robertson explains, the noradrenaline system is critical to how well focused we are in a task, how much we feel in control of what we are doing. It can help us get back to sleep, and even, according to recent studies, reduce the impact of chronic pain.

Professor Robertson calls slow, deep breathing 'the most precise pharmaceutical you could ever give yourself', with the added bonus that it is side-effect free: 'You can do it in a meeting, and no one needs to know – it works like a mini reset button for your brain.'

CASE STUDY

Mark, community investment officer

'I was keen to try deep-breathing exercises in the hope that they would help me reduce my heart rate and maintain a sense of calm and control when I'm having to deal with stressful situations at work. So I tried the 4:6 technique, breathing in for a count of four and out for a count of six for a few minutes every day for a week.

I struggled at first to get my breathing in time with the slower count, but it did get easier, especially if I stood up with my feet firmly planted on the floor and kept my eyes closed so I could focus properly. I noticed I had become a bit slouched but deep breathing helped me to subconsciously hold my shoulders back. As a result of the exercises, I have slept better and I've felt calmer – with the bonus that my posture seems to have improved too.'

Professor Robertson calls slow, deep breathing 'the most precise pharmaceutical you could ever give yourself', with the added bonus that it is side-effect free – it works like a mini reset button for your brain.

just one thing

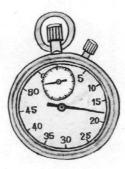

exercise less, but more often

How to do it: break your exercise up into bite-sized chunks, perhaps three lots of 10 minutes.

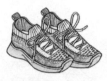

The single reason most people cite for not exercising is lack of time. And it certainly can be tricky to find the two and a half hours a week of moderately intense activity you need to meet the recommended guidelines. So why not try some 'exercise snacks'? Research shows that peppering them throughout the day can be just as good – if not better – for your health.

Indeed, squeezing just a few short periods of activity into your week can help improve your blood glucose and blood pressure more effectively than one concentrated 30-minute workout.

According to Dr Marie Murphy, who is professor of exercise and health at Ulster University, the additional benefits of exercise snacking come from the fact that your metabolism remains raised for a while after each brief bout of activity.

'The main benefit of exercise snacking is the fact that it is more likely to happen,' she says, 'and some exercise is better than no exercise at all. But building a few exercise snacks into your day can be more beneficial than one single exercise session because when we stop exercising our metabolism keeps going a bit quicker for a while as we recover. So three 10-minute snacks probably add up to a greater energy expenditure than one 30-minute session.'

Studies show exercise snacking is great for cardiovascular fitness, helping to lower blood pressure and cholesterol levels, as well as reduce weight, specifically in body fat.

'Even though you might not feel as if you are doing much, it is still a great way to get your heart rate up, and your circulation going,' says Professor Murphy. 'It means you're activating a lot of the enzymes that help with metabolism, which is a great way to keep blood sugar levels stable and reduce the risk of type 2 diabetes. When you contract your muscles, you activate the enzymes which allow glucose to move across from the blood into the muscle as fuel, so using big muscle groups, such as the quads (thighs) and glutes (buttocks), puts demand on your blood glucose which helps to keep levels naturally regulated,' she explains.

One small study of people with type 2 diabetes found that six minutes of brisk walking broken into one-minute chunks throughout the day was a more effective way to reduce blood sugar levels than a 30-minute walk before dinner. Better still, the exercise snackers recorded reduced blood sugar levels both on the day they did their six minute walks and for the following 24 hours.

Other studies (from Japan) have also shown that several short bouts of exercise are more effective at lowering blood pressure than one longer daily exercise session.

So what's the best way to get started with exercise snacking?

'Recent evidence suggests almost any level of activity counts,' says Professor Murphy. 'Ten-minute chunks are a good figure to aim for, but don't worry if you can only do five minutes each time. The key message is that every single minute counts and if you've only got a few minutes you can still use them wisely to contribute towards your overall activity goals.'

Better still: you don't have to get hot and sweaty and there's no need to get changed into specialist fitness gear. The aim is simply to get your heart beating harder whenever you can, doing enough 'snacks' to add up to 30 minutes of activity during the course of your day.

There's no doubt, snacking is a really easy way to fit activity into your life, particularly if you're not a great lover of exercise. The key point is that *anything* you can do is going to be far better for your health than having the intention of going to the gym, running out of time and missing out on exercise altogether.

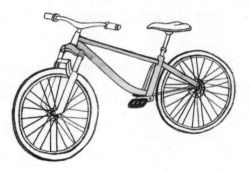

EXERCISE SNACKS TO TEMPT YOU

An exercise snack can last from just 20 seconds to 10 minutes, and it doesn't matter what you do, as long as you are elevating your heart rate and getting a bit warm.

★ You could start your day, as I do, with a brisk 10–15-minute early-morning walk.

★ At midday you could jump on your bike (or exercise bike) and pedal hard, against resistance for 20 seconds. This is known as HIIT, high-intensity interval training, and a couple of 20-second bursts really can make a difference. We live at the top of a steep hill and if I cycle into town to buy food I do a couple of 20-second bursts, where I really push myself, on the way back.

★ If that sounds a bit much, then you could try running up and down a flight of stairs two or three times.

★ Or do 60 seconds of star jumps, or jogging on the spot.

★ Whenever you're waiting for the kettle to boil, do some push-ups off the kitchen counter, or squats.

★ Take a 10-minute walk around the block at lunchtime.

★ Put on some fast upbeat music and dance enthusiastically for the length of one or two tracks (we'll come to why you might want to make dancing Just One Thing, on page 172).

★ Take large 'lunge' steps from one side of the room to the other.

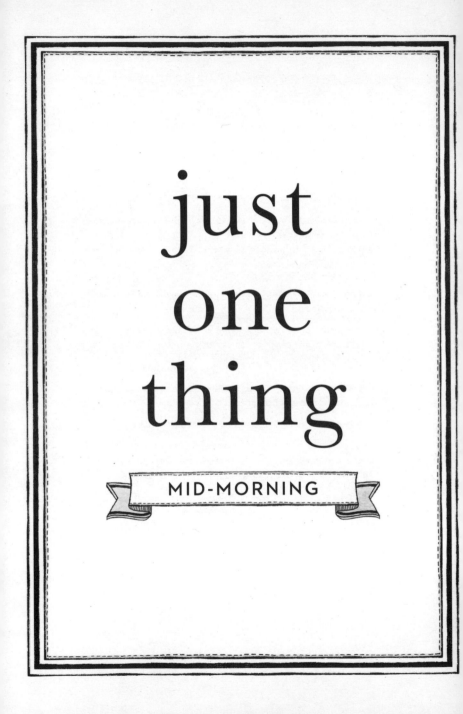

just one thing

MID-MORNING

eccentric
exercise

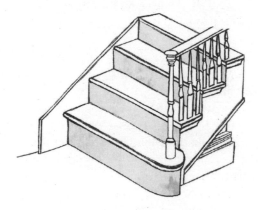

How to do it: run downhill, walk briskly down the stairs or lower weights.

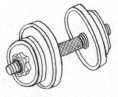

While I am on the subject of exercise, one of the best ways to get the most out of any workout is to make it 'eccentric'. You might think that running up a hill is better for you than jogging down, or that climbing a flight of stairs is going to challenge your muscles more intensively than taking the lift to the top of a tall building and walking down, but in fact, the opposite is true.

It seems crazy, but this is the new science of 'eccentric exercise', and I find it fascinating!

The name comes from the fact that contracting your muscles (to climb stairs or lift weights) is called 'concentric exercise' but any work that goes into those muscles while they are stretched and elongated (as you go downstairs or lower the weights) is known as 'eccentric exercise' (pronounced 'ee-centric').

Tony Kay is professor of biomechanics at the University of Northampton. He explains that all forms of exercise create microscopic damage to the muscles. This stimulates the release of hormones which trigger your cells to re-build that muscle stronger than before. Concentric exercises (such as bicep curls or squats) recruit and fatigue many different muscle fibres.

Although the eccentric part of the exercise (as we lower the weight, or sink down into a squat) recruits fewer fibres, it does this with a load that is up to four times higher. Which, he says, creates far greater microscopic damage to those cells and fibres.

'The greater damage means the body burns more calories in the process of repair and recovery *after* the exercise has been performed,' he says. 'This raises the metabolic rate and increases strength in a far more effective way than conventional forms of exercise.'

In one study, volunteers were randomly allocated to either walking up or down a set of stairs in a 10-storey building twice a week, and taking the lift in the other direction. Not surprisingly, both groups saw health improvements, but amazingly the group who walked down rather than up the stairs ended up with greater improvements in resting heart rate (a reliable overall measure of fitness). They also saw a greater improvement in their insulin sensitivity and blood fat levels. The group walking down also saw greater improvement in muscle function and bone density than the group walking up; in fact, the group doing what I would consider to be the easier task improved their muscle strength by 34 per cent – by twice as much as those who had to walk up the stairs each time!

In addition, the group walking down showed greater improvements in a balance test, which would lead to a reduced risk of falls and injury.

Another study comparing older adults doing traditional versus eccentric exercise found the eccentric group had a 38 per cent improvement in leg strength compared to just 8 per cent improvement in the traditional exercise group.

Other studies have shown the benefits of eccentric exercise in young, healthy male footballers (such as dramatic increases in strength), as well as in over-65s (who showed 30–50 per cent increases in strength and a 10 per cent increase in muscle mass in just six weeks.) 'The effects are far, far greater than we would expect from normal exercise,' he concludes.

This is really impressive and completely counterintuitive. And it turns out that any exercise that requires you to lengthen your muscles under resistance will have the same beneficial effect – whether it is running downhill or slowly lowering yourself down into a squat or a press-up. The way it works is that when you are going down, the muscles in your legs or arms lengthen to slow the pace of descent. Similarly, when you are lowering a set of weights, the muscles lengthen and have to work harder to protect your body from damage.

Professor Kay says both yoga and pilates incorporate poses which require you to slowly lower yourself, thereby causing an eccentric contraction, which will 'increase flexibility, muscle mass, bone density and strength'.

Do them right and not only will eccentric exercises keep you in good shape but they will also help your body to continue burning calories after you have finished – more so than a seemingly 'tougher' workout. This could be the metabolic secret that has been hiding in your workout all along!

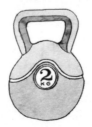

You might think that running up a hill is better for you than jogging down, or that climbing a flight of stairs is going to challenge your muscles more intensively than taking the lift to the top of a tall building and walking down, but in fact, the opposite is true.

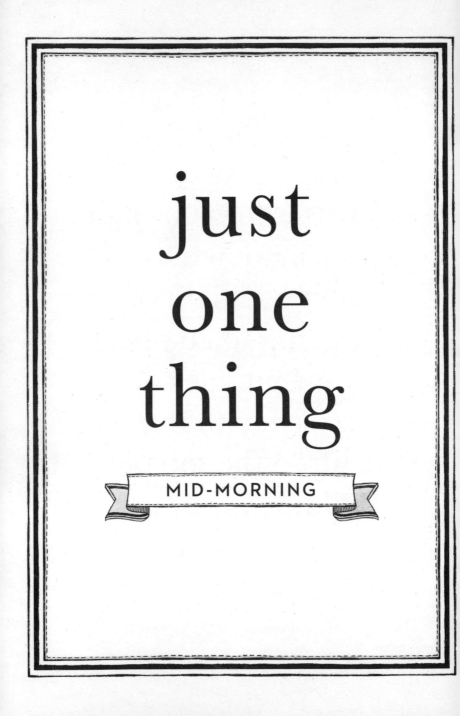

just
one
thing

MID-MORNING

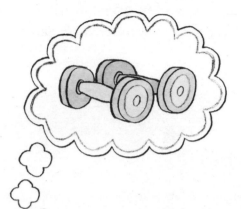

think
yourself
stronger

How to do it: spend 15–20 minutes a day mentally rehearsing a skill or activity you'd like to perfect.

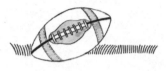

I've written quite a bit so far about the benefits of getting more active. This might mean going for early-morning walks (page 44), doing intelligent exercises (page 16) and making them eccentric (page 100).

But surprisingly enough, there is research that shows that simply *thinking* about doing a physical activity or playing a sport can increase your muscle strength and boost your performance.

You might have heard rugby players talk about mentally rehearsing the ball flying through the goal posts before they take a kick, or runners on the starting blocks imagining themselves speeding around the track. Elite athletes have long used a technique called 'motor imagery' in which they imagine themselves performing successfully, and there is evidence that this really can increase their chance of doing so.

Motor imagery can also boost performance in other areas of life, from surgery to music. Studies have shown that surgeons perform better if they mentally rehearse an operation before they actually do it, while some professional musicians find they benefit from mentally practising their instrument, as well as actually playing it.

Dr Helen O'Shea, a cognitive psychologist at University of Limerick, explains how it works: 'When you really focus on an action or imagine you are performing a movement, you'll be sending those really focused signals to the relevant parts of your body.'

In 1990, researchers from Louisiana State University asked women to imagine extending their knee and contracting their thigh muscle in five-second bursts. At the end of the study, the strength in their thigh muscles had increased by 12.6 per cent.

When a team I was working with conducted a similar experiment, we found muscle strength increased by 8 per cent. The muscles didn't actually get bigger, but it seems the volunteers were able to activate 20 per cent more muscle fibre having mentally rehearsed the action.

'Although the muscles involved won't grow, the drive towards those muscles becomes much more fine-tuned, so you end up only using the muscles that are key for that movement and not wasting any energy on muscles that are not,' explains Dr O'Shea.

'We know that motor imagery can improve our accuracy, our speed, our strength,' she says, 'and we have found it actually alters the way our brain operates too.'

'Unfortunately, you can't use it to boost fitness levels,' she adds. 'For motor imagery to work, you need to be familiar with the physical movement first; only then can you use your imagination to prime your motor systems so that when you come to actually execute the movement everything is finely tuned and ready to go.'

DR O'SHEA'S RECOMMENDATIONS
FOR PERFORMANCE ENHANCING

★ The effect is more powerful if you perform your motor imagery at the same place you would be doing the activity (the football pitch, the tennis court, the golf course), as location helps you form a really vivid and accurate mental representation of the movement.

★ Ideally wear the same clothes and carry the same kit you'd normally use.

★ Try to feel your body perform the action in your mind (scoring a goal, serving an ace, hitting the perfect putt), keeping the same flow and pace as when you physically execute that action.

★ Keep your eyes open as you visualise the impact of your imagined actions and a successful conclusion and aim to get as close as possible to that feeling of success.

★ Alternate four sessions of motor imagery with one physical execution, then go back to the motor imagery.

CASE STUDY
Tom

'I'm the goalkeeper with a five-a-side football team but I'm keen to try my skills as a striker. I'm definitely out of practice – it must be 18 years since I last scored a goal! I admit I did feel a little foolish standing in the garden dressed in my sports kit, holding a football and imagining myself kicking it straight into the goal, but I let my imagination go wild and occasionally added in images of the goalie floundering and the roar of the crowd...

I have no idea if the mental practice actually helped create that connection between my brain and my muscles, but I can report that I did score two goals in two games. Admittedly, I missed a host of chances, but not by much. I felt a lot more confident with the ball at my feet.'

Elite athletes have long used a technique called 'motor imagery' in which they imagine themselves performing successfully, and there is evidence that this really can increase their chance of doing so.

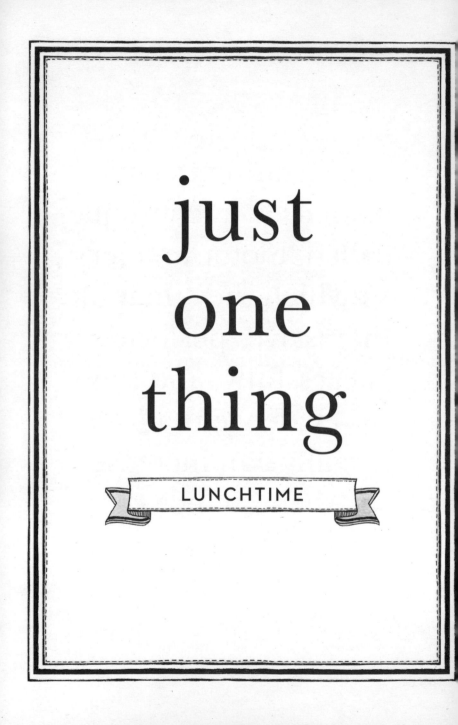

just
one
thing

LUNCHTIME

enjoy oily fish

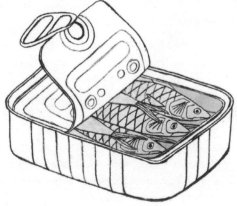

How to do it: eat a portion of mackerel, salmon, sardines, herring or anchovies at least twice a week.

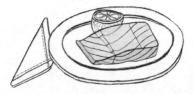

These days, one of the foods I really enjoy eating, whether for breakfast, lunch or my evening meal, is oily fish. If you had told me this 30 years ago, I would have been astonished. Growing up, I used to hate fish. Too often it was served overcooked or watery or submerged in some gloopy sauce. But these days we eat oily fish at least three times a week, and usually far more often. As well as being tasty and wonderfully simple to prepare, oily fish is a really great source of protein and omega 3 fatty acids, which have been shown to be great for reducing chronic inflammation. Which in turn means a reduced risk of heart disease and depression.

When it comes to topping up your omega 3 levels, the *kind* of fish matters: white fish, such as cod, might be a good source of protein and other nutrients, but it is low in omega 3. And tinned tuna doesn't count as an oily fish either. So what should you eat?

Think SMASH:

Salmon
Mackerel
Anchovies
Sardines
Herring

It really is worth adding oily fish to your regular diet – and always look out for sustainable sources. The best proven benefits come from its impact on heart health, but eating oily fish has also been shown to reduce your risk of cancer and dementia, as well as being good for your joints.

And is oily fish a good brain food, as my mother always used to claim? Yes it is. Fish-eaters have been shown to have larger brains – particularly frontal lobes, an area important for focus, and temporal lobes, an area crucial for memory, learning and cognition. Other studies show that consuming omega 3 can boost working memory, planning and focus – and even verbal fluency. And it's not just your brain performance – scientists have recently found that it improves mood and reduces symptoms of depression.

So, what's actually going on? Dr Simon Dyall, a nutritional neuroscientist at the University of Roehampton, explains that omega 3s are made up of fatty acids called EPA and DHA. 'DHA is the one that appears beneficial in ageing. Whereas interestingly, in mood, EPA appears more beneficial,' he says. 'We also know they have an important role in turning off inflammation, and both dementia and ageing have a very high inflammation component.'

The fact that oily fish is so good at reducing chronic inflammation is one of the reasons why eating plenty of it can also reduce joint pain and may even protect against the negative effects of air pollution on your skin, heart and blood fat levels.

Simon is a big fan of fish – and now I am too! Experts recommend eating oily fish rather than taking a supplement, but if you're vegan or vegetarian, omega 3 supplements, which are produced from algae, are a good alternative, and fish oils can be helpful if you really hate the taste of fish.

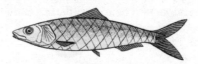

Is oily fish a good brain food, as my mother always used to claim? Yes, it is. Studies show that consuming omega 3 can boost working memory, planning and focus – and even verbal fluency.

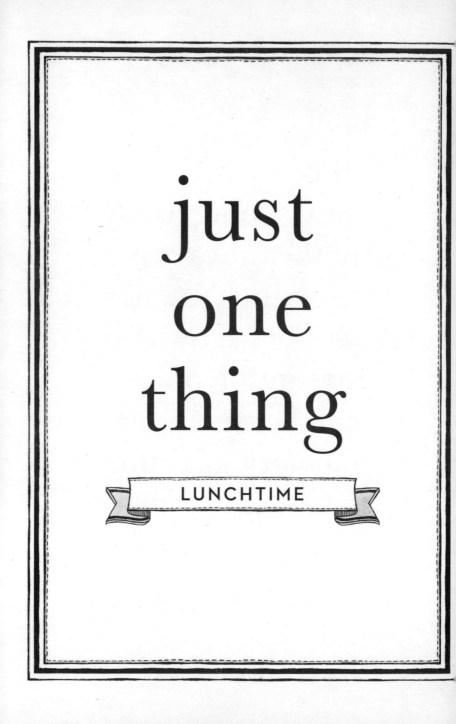

just one thing

LUNCHTIME

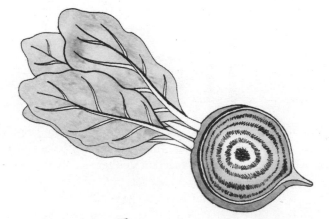

eat beetroot

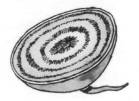

How to do it: eat two to three beetroot two to three times a week.

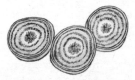

You might think of beetroot as a slightly old-fashioned and earthy-tasting root vegetable – which it is – but I am impressed by research that shows that consuming this vegetable, either as a shot (you can buy concentrated beetroot juice in bottles) or as part of a salad, can have impressive effects on your body. It has been shown to improve physical and cognitive performance and keep your heart healthy, and may even help you run faster.

Beetroots are an intense purply-pink colour, which is a tell-tale sign of powerful antioxidants called betalains, which help fight the ravages of age and have been shown (in laboratory studies) to kill colon cancer cells.

But the real secret to beetroot is the fact that it is incredibly rich in nitrates. Nitrates have acquired a bad name because they are often added to preserved meats such as bacon, ham and salami, and studies show that eating too much of these products could increase your risk of bowel cancer.

But when we consume nitrate-rich vegetables such as beetroot, something remarkable happens. Bacteria naturally living in our mouths change that nitrate into a chemical called a nitr*ite*. This compound is then changed by other processes in the body into nitric oxide, which helps to dilate blood vessels and increase blood flow to muscles, organs and the brain.

One of the ways in which Viagra – the famous little blue pill that helps ageing men perform sexually – works is by triggering the release of nitric oxide. It is no coincidence that the Romans believed beetroot juice was a powerful aphrodisiac.

Andy Jones, professor of applied physiology at the University of Exeter, is mainly interested in the impact that beetroots have on endurance and sporting performance. In one of his early studies, he asked a group of men, aged 19 to 38, to drink either beetroot juice or a placebo (blackcurrant juice) for six days, before completing a series of gruelling tests on an exercise bike. Then they swapped over.

When the group drank the beetroot juice they were able to cycle for an average of 11.25 minutes afterwards, which was 92 seconds longer than when they were given the placebo.

In another study, Professor Jones asked a group of competitive cyclists to complete a series of time trials, covering 16km, after drinking beetroot juice. What they didn't know was that on one occasion they had normal beetroot juice, while on the other the beetroot juice had had the nitrate removed. The cyclists were, on average, 45 seconds faster when they were nitrate-powered, which in a competition would be significant.

The beneficial effect of beetroot is most pronounced if you favour high-intensity workouts, as I do. 'We found volunteers eating beetroot a couple of hours before an intense bout of exercise were able to keep going for as much as 16 per cent longer than those who didn't eat beetroot,' he says. 'As a result of our study, beetroot was a massive hit with athletes at the 2012 Olympic games in London – nearly every athlete was sipping beetroot juice!'

The beetroot-fuelled increase in nitric oxide not only means your blood vessels dilate, allowing more oxygen to reach your muscles, but also makes your muscles more efficient.

The same beneficial effect seems to apply to your heart and brain. Studies have shown that beetroot juice can improve reaction times in older but active adults, and it also has the potential to reduce the risk of our biggest killers, stroke.

'Nitric oxide is a vasodilator which causes blood vessels to widen and allow more blood flow to our tissues,' explains Professor Jones. 'This can be enough to lower blood pressure to such an extent that it reduces the possibility of cardiac event and strokes.'

A few years ago, I took part in a small study with Professor Jones in which we asked a group of volunteers with raised blood pressure to spend a few weeks feasting on a diet rich in beetroot. This led to a fall in average blood pressure in the group of about 5mmHg, which, if maintained, would translate into a reduction in their risk of stroke and heart attack of about 10 per cent. This is in line with other randomised clinical trials.

Professor Jones says the optimal time to eat your beetroot is two to three hours before you hit the gym. 'That's because it takes a bit of time for the body to process the nitrate. We do rely on the bacteria in our mouths to make this conversion for us, and this takes time.'

Most studies have been done with people sipping daily shots of beetroot juice. But Professor Jones suggests that just by adding a little beetroot to your diet on a regular basis you can keep your nitrite levels topped up: 'Our ability to produce nitric oxide naturally gets worse as we get older, which is one reason why blood pressure tends to rise with age, so one way to offset this decline might be to supplement with nitrate from our diet,' he says. Be warned, though: beetroot will turn your wee pink!

HOW TO CONSUME MORE BEETROOT

The nitrate content in pickled and most vacuum-packed pre-cooked beetroot is typically low, so buying it raw or growing your own is best. Nitrates are water-soluble, which means if you tip away the cooking liquid after boiling beetroot you could be throwing away a lot of the nitrates. Try roasting or baking it rather than boiling it – that way you will retain more of the nitrates.

★ Top and tail fresh beetroot, wrap in foil and then roast in the oven for 40–50 minutes, perhaps when you are cooking something else. They are cooked when a fork can easily slide in. Enjoy them hot or cold, as a side dish or cubed in salads.

★ Grate raw beetroot into a pink coleslaw or sauerkraut (I'd recommend you wear gloves to avoid staining your fingers).

★ Whizz raw or cooked beetroot into a smoothie with an apple.

★ Juice it with a spritz of fresh lemon juice.

★ Buy beetroot juice (look for unsweetened varieties).

★ You can even grate beetroot into cakes. Indeed, you will find some delicious beet-related recipes (including beetroot brownies) on my wife Dr Clare Bailey's Instagram account: Instagram.com/drclarebailey.

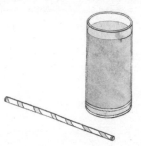

just one thing

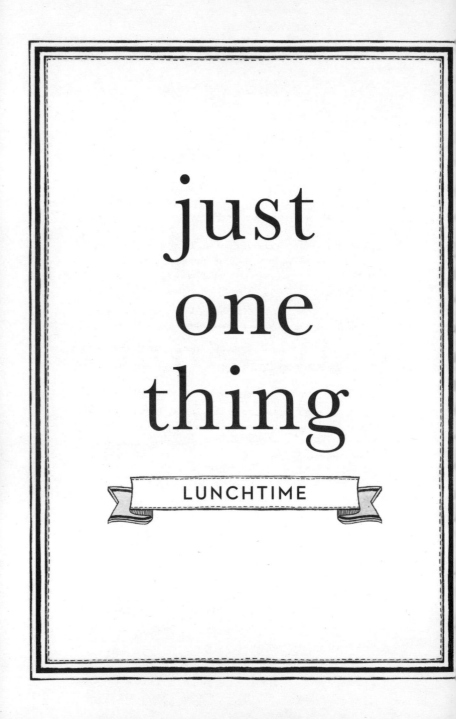

LUNCHTIME

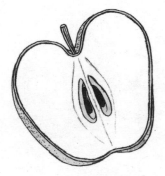

an apple
a day

How to do it: eat an apple, unpeeled, every day.

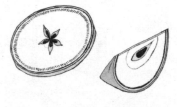

When I have lunch, whether it is some oily fish or a sandwich on the go, I like to finish with an apple. I love the flavour and I find it clears the palate. Apples are also my go-to dessert, whether as apple crumble, baked apple or apple cake.

So I'm delighted to be able to tell you that there really is a lot of truth in the old saying that 'an apple a day keeps the doctor away'.

Dr Catherine Bondonno is a nutritionist at the Institute for Nutrition Research at Edith Cowan University in Western Australia and she told me that, as well as containing lots of fibre, apples are rich in beneficial compounds called flavonoids.

'Flavonoids are produced by plants to protect them from sunlight and disease, and it is thought they have a similarly protective effect in humans when we eat them,' Dr Bondonno explains. 'Research has shown that flavonoids from fruit can increase the production of a molecule in our body called nitric oxide that regulates blood pressure and maintains blood vessel health.'

As we have just seen in the Just One Thing on beetroot, nitric oxide has multiple health benefits.

Most of an apple's flavonoids lurk in or just under the skin – so ideally you should eat your apples unpeeled to gain the maximum benefits.

'Eating flavonoids *with* fibre changes the way our bodies break down and absorb the flavonoid compounds,' she told me. 'It means the flavonoids pass through the small intestine to reach the large intestine, where helpful bacteria break them down into compounds called phenolic acids which help to reduce inflammation and improve blood pressure.

'Working in tandem, flavonoids and fibre appear to increase the quantity of beneficial bacteria and decrease the quantity of harmful bacteria residing in our gut,' she adds.

Dr Bondonno says that, along with reducing inflammation and improving blood pressure, apples have been shown to lower cholesterol and reduce the risk of diabetes, and that they contain other nutrients such as vitamins C and K, plus minerals like copper and potassium which boost their health-giving properties further.

In one study she was involved with, where for 15 years they followed a large group of women, all of whom were over the age of 70 at the outset, they found that those who ate at least one apple a day were 35 per cent less likely to die over that time than those who shunned apples.

Apples could also help you maintain your weight. One US study found that middle-aged women asked to eat 75g of dried apple a day not only reduced their LDL (bad cholesterol) levels by 23 per cent, but despite the extra calories, they actually lost 1.5kg – just over 3lb – in weight too.

Although peeling your apples is a no-no, you can cook them without destroying the beneficial compounds, which appear to last well, even if they have been in storage for some time. And if you are interested in which varieties are best, well, Dr Bondonno has tested a range of them and found the ones with the highest concentration of flavonoids are Pink Ladies.

I enjoy apples as a snack, chopped up in my yoghurt for breakfast and baked as a pudding. Why don't you try to make them a regular part of your diet?

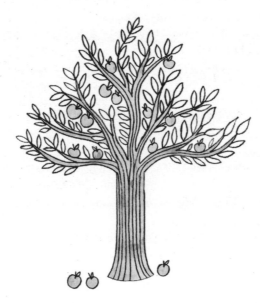

Working in tandem, flavonoids and fibre appear to increase the quantity of beneficial bacteria and decrease the quantity of harmful bacteria residing in our gut.

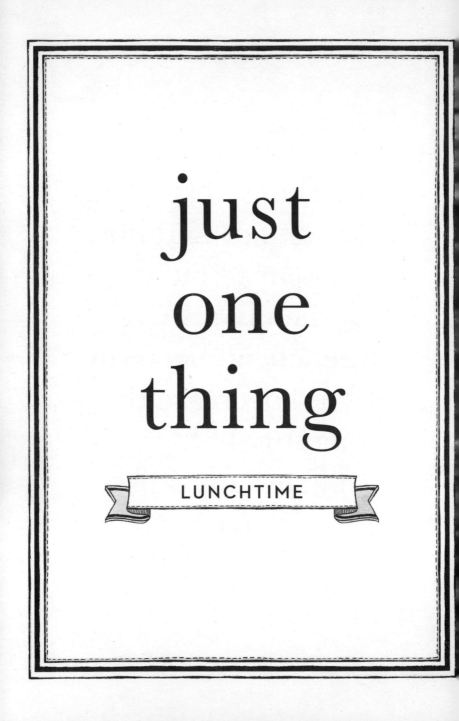

just one thing

LUNCHTIME

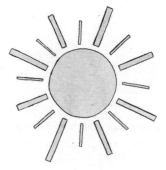

get some sun

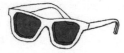

How to do it: roll up your sleeves and your trouser legs and sit in the sun for 10–45 minutes, depending on how dark your skin is.

For years we have been warned that excessive sun exposure puts us at risk of skin cancers and premature skin ageing, which is true. But more recent research suggests that a short blast of sunshine each day during the spring and summer months could be very good for us indeed – lifting mood, lowering blood pressure and keeping our immune system in good shape. And if you're careful not to burn, the benefits should outweigh any risks.

One of the well-known benefits of getting more sun is that it will boost your levels of vitamin D. Although you can get some vitamin D from foods such as oily fish and egg yolks, unless you eat a LOT of fish you need to look for other sources. Luckily, the skin is a vitamin D factory which takes free sunlight and transforms it into this amazing nutrient. When the sunlight falls on your skin, it hits a molecule in it, changing it into 'pre-vitamin D', which is then converted into vitamin D over the next few hours.

As well as being vital for strong bones, vitamin D contributes to a well-functioning immune system. Studies have shown that people with very low vitamin D are also at greater risk of heart disease, dementia, diabetes and multiple sclerosis – even some forms of cancer.

According to Ann Webb, professor of atmospheric radiation at Manchester University, daily exposure to sunlight during the spring and summer months should help you avoid vitamin D deficiency, though if you live in the northern hemisphere, you will probably need to take a supplement during the winter months (October to March), when the sun isn't very strong. At that time of year, you'd have to spend much longer, with more skin exposed, to get the same effect. I suspect few of us would want to sit semi-naked outdoors during the winter months just to boost our vitamin D…

Professor Webb told me that during the spring and summer, 'little and often' is the best approach and that if you have fair skin, 10–15 minutes of sunlight exposure should be enough for unprotected skin. People with darker skin should aim for 25–40 minutes because dark skin has more melanin: this is a natural sunscreen, but it also hinders the skin's ability to absorb vitamin D.

Simply holding your face up to the sun probably won't be enough – so roll up your sleeves and trouser legs if you can.

If you live somewhere really hot, it is best to avoid going out at midday, but in cooler climates, like the UK's, you get most bang for your buck in the middle of the day when the sun is strongest.

There are, of course, other benefits to being out in the sun than just generating vitamin D. As we discovered earlier (see page 45), sunlight is important for resetting our internal clocks – which is important for people who, like me, experience seasonal affective disorder (SAD).

Sunlight triggers the release of serotonin, which is a natural mood-booster that is deficient in people with SAD.

On top of that, sunlight can also help lower our blood pressure.

Scientists from Edinburgh University have shown that 20 minutes of sun on an arm is enough to boost production of nitric oxide, which causes blood vessels to expand and consequently brings our blood pressure down.

So don't shun the sun! Used wisely, it is a truly life-enhancing thing.

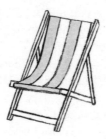

CASE STUDY

Mehreen, teacher and TV presenter

Mehreen had been diagnosed with low levels of vitamin D, after complaining of feeling tired, heavy and lethargic. But simply going outside every day between 12 and 2pm changed everything: 'I love the sun! it makes me feel really happy. After just 10 minutes outside I feel relaxed and lighter. It's great to know I'm topping up on vitamin D, but I've found it is a refreshing mental break which benefits me psychologically too.'

HOW LONG SHOULD YOU SIT IN THE SUN?

The amount of time you can safely spend outside will depend on your skin type – darker skins absorb vitamin D more slowly. It is also important to be aware that some medication (such as antibiotics) and skin products (such as retinol) can increase skin sensitivity. Whatever your skin type, it's important to seek cover or put on sunscreen before you start to burn.

Pale Northern European skin – 10–15 mins
Darker South Asian and Afro-Caribbean skin – 25–40 mins

just one thing

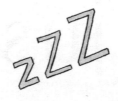

take a nap

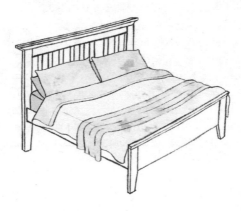

How to do it: snatch the chance for a 20-minute snooze after lunch.

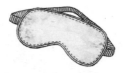

If, like me, you are a poor sleeper and often suffer from a mid-afternoon slump, instead of grabbing a tea or coffee, why not take advantage of this dip in energy to have a little shut-eye?

You'll be in good company – British prime minister Winston Churchill regularly recharged himself with an afternoon nap, writing in his memoirs that 'even if it only lasts 20 minutes, it is sufficient to renew all the vital forces'.

He was clearly on to something because recent research suggests that a nap can do wonderful things for your mind and your body.

Not only can napping boost mood and wellbeing, but large studies have even shown a link between regular napping and good heart health. One study found an occasional daytime nap was associated with a 48 per cent lower risk of heart attack, stroke or heart failure – if there was a pill powerful enough to do that the manufacturers would make a fortune!

If you (or your boss) are worried that an afternoon snooze is a bit self-indulgent, then you might like to know it can improve your thinking skills too. Studies show napping can improve your performance in tests and strengthen your capacity to learn if you don't routinely get enough sleep at night and be more beneficial than tacking on an extra 30 minutes' sleep during the night.

Dr Sarah Mednick, a cognitive neuroscientist and sleep researcher at the University of California, is a big fan: 'Our research shows that a good nap can produce the same benefits as a full night of sleep,' she says. 'It can be a great way to ease the stress and anxiety caused by insufficient sleep, helping you to regulate emotions.'

Her team's research shows any rest longer than five minutes can be helpful, with different lengths of nap time conferring different benefits. 'When you first drop off, you typically go into stage one sleep for two or three minutes before moving into stage two sleep, which is great for enhancing attention, memory and motor skills,' she explains.

'A 20-minute nap is a useful way to push the reset button, increasing alertness and attention as well as sharpening motor skills (particularly if you need to perform a task which requires co-ordinated muscle movements).'

A 60-minute nap gives you enough time to move into a stage called 'slow-wave' sleep which, according to Dr Mednick, can help to enhance memory: 'Slow-wave sleep is like a "cardiovascular holiday" which gives your entire system the chance to calm down, and for your body to recuperate its resources, to recover from the stress of the day,' she says.

A 90-minute nap, particularly taken in the morning, gives you access to REM (rapid eye movement) sleep. 'There's a lot of evidence that this enhances a creative state of mind because the frontal lobe of your brain shuts down, allowing for freewheeling connections in the brain.'

The downside of a long nap – anything lasting more than 30 minutes – is that it may well reduce your sleep drive and you may then find it harder to get to sleep when you stagger to bed in the evening. So most of the experts I spoke to suggested that

20–30 minutes was the optimum length of time. And try to take it in the early afternoon, soon after lunch – no later than 3pm – as a late-afternoon nap can interfere with night-time sleep.

CASE STUDY

Caroline, mental health specialist

Caroline gets up at 5am every day to exercise and then juggle the challenges of work and being mum to three young children. She says: 'My sleep is often broken and I spend much of my day feeling tired – I'm usually shattered at 2–3pm – but I just crack on. The idea of a snooze seems too self-indulgent. I've always got too much else to do to give having a nap any kind of priority.

When I first tried it, I found it hard to fall asleep, possibly because it's not my normal routine, although it does feel rather lovely to lie down and rest, even if I don't drop off. However, I've gradually got better at being able to fall asleep straight away – an eye mask certainly helps and I've definitely noticed an improvement in my productivity in the afternoons. After a bad night's sleep, everything seems like a battle, but when I can get a nap things seem more breezy. In fact, sometimes it really is quite magical – it feels like I'm giving myself a well-deserved break!'

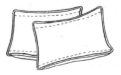

If you (or your boss) are worried that an afternoon snooze is a bit self-indulgent, then you might like to know that not only is a short nap good for your heart health, but it can improve your thinking skills too.

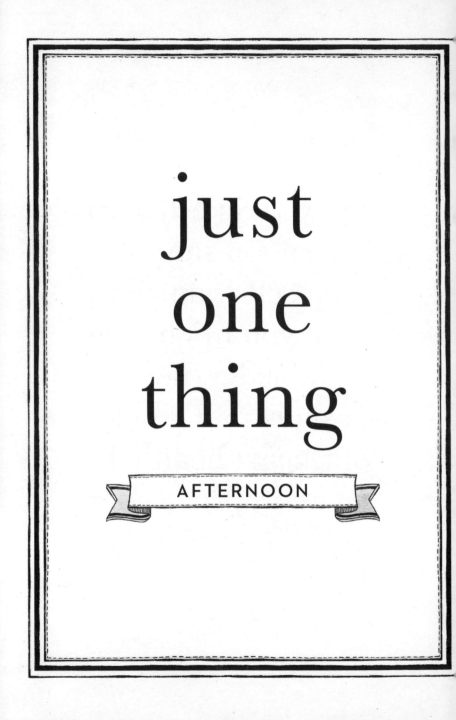

just
one
thing

AFTERNOON

get some house plants

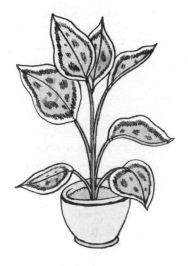

How to do it: put five fast-growing plants in the rooms you use most often.

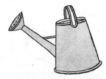

My office at home is where I spend a lot of time. It has always been a rather bland and functional room, but recently I've taken to filling it with plants. I've chosen very hardy species like aspidistra (which are almost unkillable), spider plants (ditto) and snake plants. They have added some much-needed life to the room, and to me.

I don't have particularly green fingers and I know nothing about horticulture, but I do like plants and I am really interested in research that suggests that house plants can boost memory, productivity, mood and even reduce indoor air pollution – plus, of course, they do look lovely.

My interest in the power of house plants was first piqued by the NASA Clean Air Study conducted in 1989 by NASA scientists who were keen to investigate ways to improve the living conditions for astronauts in space. They showed that by putting certain plants in an enclosed space they could reduce the amount of volatile organic compounds (VOCs) in the air. VOCs are chemicals that are typically released into the air by building materials, aerosol sprays and cleaning products. One VOC, limonene, is often added to cleaning products to give a citrusy scent, but it can react with ozone in the air to form an unpleasant substance called formaldehyde, which is traditionally used to preserve corpses.

Some people are more sensitive than others, but according to the American Lung Association, 'VOCs can irritate the eyes, nose and throat, can cause difficulty breathing and nausea, and can damage the central nervous system as well as other organs.' They are a recognised cause of 'sick building syndrome'.

If you search online for 'NASA Clean Air Study', you will find the sort of plants they tested, but among their top 10 were English ivy, devil's ivy, peace lily, Chinese evergreen and variegated sansevieria (snake plant).

If you live in a drafty house or a well-ventilated office, you probably don't have a problem. But many modern houses and offices can have quite high levels of VOCs because they are sealed to save energy. The level will depend on how well ventilated the room is and how many VOC-releasing products you use. But it may also depend on how many house plants you have.

In 2006, when researchers from the Plants and Environmental Quality Group in Australia did a study in which they put house plants in 60 offices with high levels of VOCs, they found the plants swiftly reduced the levels by between 60 and 75 per cent. They concluded that 'potted plants can provide an efficient, self-regulating, low-cost and sustainable way of dealing with indoor air pollution.'

But do they really improve health? In another study, Norwegian researchers assessed the impact of introducing plants in an office, a school and a hospital radiology department. When the office was filled with plants, people reported fewer coughs, headaches and fatigue. The researchers noted a similar reduction in health-related complaints in the hospital and school.

And thanks to the fact that, during the day, they absorb carbon dioxide and breathe out oxygen, plants can also reduce carbon dioxide levels and boost humidity – two things that make us humans feel better. High levels of carbon dioxide can make you lightheaded or give you a headache and this can impair thinking and decision making.

Whether it is thanks to improved air quality, or just the pleasure we get from having nature all around us, there is good evidence that plants have a positive effect on wellbeing, focus and concentration.

Dr Tijana Blanusa from the University of Reading is principal horticultural scientist for the Royal Horticultural Society and has spent years researching the impact of house plants on humans. Her studies show that having plants in the office has an overwhelmingly positive effect. In one study, which involved introducing plants and then taking them away again, she found that people reported more stress and reduced efficiency and attention after the plants were removed.

'If you have a massive problem at work or at home, no amount of house plants will fix it for you,' she adds, 'but when it comes to small everyday life tasks, plants have a positive role to play.'

CASE STUDY

Davinia from Belfast has a home full of house plants, but she told me her office is a bleak, plant-free zone. So I asked her to bring four plants in from home and put them on her desk and then monitor her mood, productivity and sleep patterns over a week. 'After just three days, I noticed I was feeling much happier at work. I found I had to break off from whatever I was doing every so often to water the plants, which I think gave my brain a break (see 'take a break', page 82). I've also noticed colleagues are popping into my office to comment on how beautiful the plants look, and we are chatting more. The extra green in my office brightens up my day and makes me happier. I'm planning to bring more plants in and create a little tropical garden in here.'

WHICH PLANTS?

Dr Blanusa says you need five or six plants in a room to really have an impact. The fast-growing, thirsty, 'physiologically active' plants tend to provide the most benefits, for example, peace lily and devil's ivy. Although succulents and cacti might be great starter plants because they are so easy to look after, she says they generally provide few benefits because they have a more limited 'gas exchange'.

She also says you can boost the benefits by keeping your plants where they have access to high levels of light: 'The more light you can give them, the better they will perform.'

★ **Mother-in-law's tongue** (also known as snake plant or sansevieria, has long elegantly spikey leaves)

★ **Spider plant** (extremely forgiving and easy to keep)

★ **Ivy**

★ **Peace lily**

★ **Aloe vera** (elegant green spikes with narrow green fleshy leaves)

★ **Rosemary** (which is a lovely herb to cook with; rub a few needles between your fingers and inhale the delicious aroma)

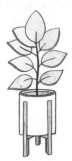

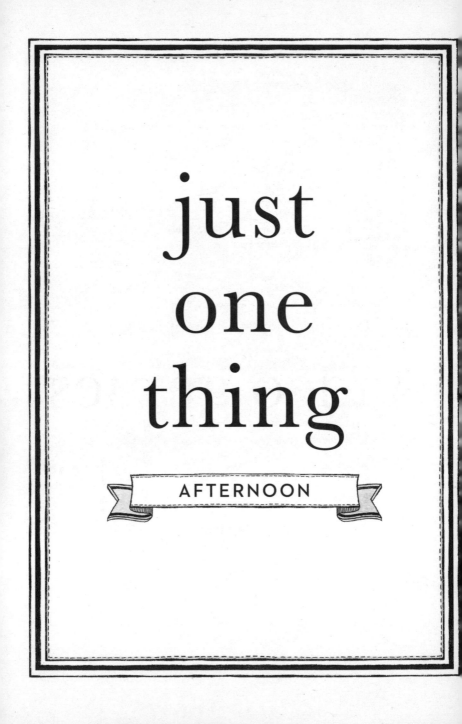

just one thing

AFTERNOON

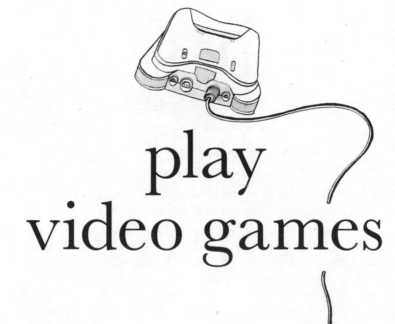

play
video games

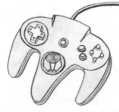

How to do it: play a high-action game for 30 minutes a day.

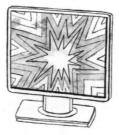

My three sons spent a large chunk of their teenage years playing video games, something that my daughter had no interest in. Funny that. I always thought that playing video games was a monumental waste of time. Like most parents, I also saw these games as horribly addictive, bad for your eyes and bad for your attention span. But, as much as I may hate to admit it, I was wrong.

Recent research suggests that action-packed gaming can be good for your brain and even for your eyesight. Games have been shown to boost your working memory (your ability to remember more than one thing at a time), your focus and your ability to multitask. There is some evidence that they can even change areas of the brain related to abstract reasoning and problem solving.

Cognitive neuroscientist Daphne Bavelier is a professor at the University of Geneva and a specialist in the impact of video games on behaviour. 'As a mum of three children, I share your concerns about video games being bad for you, but as a scientist I have been pleasantly surprised to see how some video games can have a positive effect on the brain and behaviour,' she says.

'The right games really can enhance how well you pay attention; they also improve perception (how well you see and hear) and show marked improvement in special cognition and working memory and the ability to multitask. We believe gaming really can make the brain more efficient at processing information.'

The games that provide the strongest cognitive benefits appear to be action games that involve quick decision making, navigating around environments and finding visual targets. These kinds of games have been shown to increase grey matter in an area associated with abstract reasoning and problem solving. 'We noticed that people who play high-paced action video games tend to perform extremely well on our tests of attention – and the effect is particularly pronounced in people who play "shooter" games rather than participation or puzzle games,' says Professor Bavelier.

It seems gaming makes you better at taking in multiple things at once, ignoring distractions and spotting details in busy, confusing scenes. These kinds of skills are, of course, useful in life as well as for killing aliens.

But what about the dark side of video games? The manufacturers use all kinds of tricks to keep you playing longer. The games can be addictive: the more you play the more you want to play. But studies have shown that they don't necessarily incite aggressive or violent behaviour as previously suspected.

Nor do they appear to be bad for your eyes. Professor Bavelier says young gamers appear to have superior eyesight. In fact, one study found that spending an hour a day on action games actually improved a form of vision called 'contrast sensitivity'. This is your ability to distinguish between shades of grey, and it naturally gets worse as we get older.

So am I too old to try gaming? Professor Bavelier recommends that older adults like me, who are new to gaming, start with driving games: 'Any game where you need to aim at a path but at the same time avoid distraction and obstacles and also collect points will help to enhance attention and attention control,' she says.

And her studies show that, if you play for 30 minutes a day, five days a week, you should see cognitive improvements in around three months.

Gaming crib sheet: sound like a pro by peppering your gaming conversation with the following terms:

★ 'They're flanking' – an opponent is trying to attack you from a different angle.

★ 'Hop on' – you are being invited to join someone's group.

★ 'In the lobby' – the waiting room where competitors assemble before a game starts.

★ 'The party' – the group of players who will be playing the game together.

★ 'I downed them' – you successfully hit an opponent.

★ 'He spawned' – the character was reborn (effectively rose from the dead).

★ 'I'm a noob' – new to the game/unfamiliar with the game.

★ 'They're on a streak' – enjoying a run of successful kills/wins.

★ 'They've been sniped' – when someone is hit by a long-distance rifle.

It seems gaming makes you better at taking in multiple things at once, ignoring distractions and spotting details in busy, confusing scenes. These kinds of skills are, of course, useful in life as well as for killing aliens.

just
one
thing

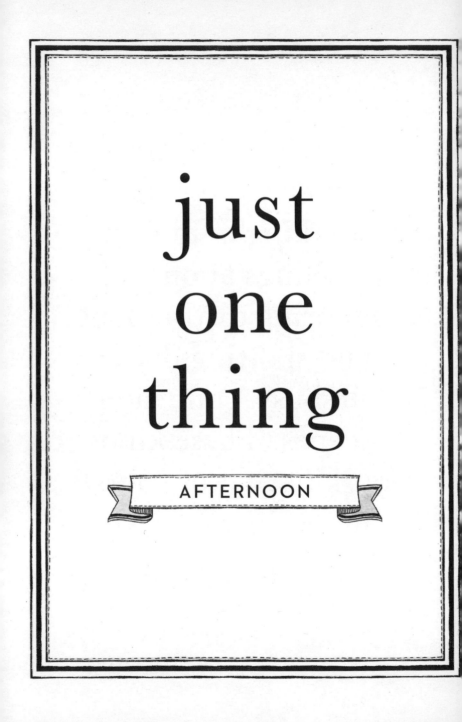

AFTERNOON

green
spaces

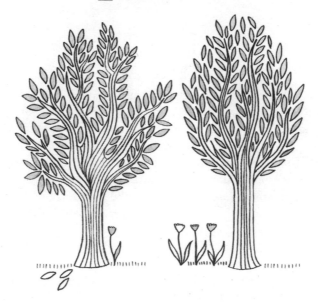

How to do it: aim to spend a few hours each week in a green space, enjoying the sights, sounds and smells.

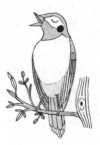

Clare and I are lucky enough to live near a wood and on the edge of lots of easily accessible countryside. Which means that in the afternoon I'm able to get away from the computer and spend some time in nature. It is great to just stop, look around, breathe in the smell of the trees, listen to the sounds of birds and appreciate the pattern of light passing through the leaves. Pausing to listen and notice your environment in this way shifts your focus outwards, makes you more engaged in the world around you and less in your own thoughts.

There are now plenty of studies showing that just being in green spaces can help reduce stress and anxiety. Not only that, but surprisingly it seems it can help boost your immune system too. The evidence is so convincing that in Scotland doctors have started to prescribe it to their patients, while in Japan, they have created a tradition of 'forest bathing' or 'having a forest shower'.

To get maximum benefit, you should aim to connect with ALL your senses: listening, inhaling, sniffing, touching and really looking at the world around you. There are some specific benefits to taking deep breaths when you are in a wood. That's because you will be inhaling phytoncides – the 'essential oils' given off by trees. These organic chemicals are created by the trees to protect themselves from microbes and insects, but they have also been shown to enhance mood and bolster your immune system.

'Spending time in a green space has two main effects on the immune system,' Professor Ming Kuo, who is director of the University of Illinois Landscape and Human Health Laboratory, told me. 'It calms what needs calming and strengthens what needs strengthening.

'Nature calms our system of inflammatory cytokines which are the alarm bells for the body. When they get overexcited, the body will mount a defence, called a cytokine storm, which can be deadly – particularly if you get a disease like Covid.

'But nature also strengthens our immunity apparatus by improving the number of natural "killer cells" in our system – and it is their job to fight viruses.' In fact, research has found that spending time in nature can increase the number of natural killer cells by up to 50 per cent, and reduce inflammatory cytokines by the same amount.'

In other words, spending time in green spaces not only keeps our immune system tuned up and strong, but also ensures that it doesn't overreact.

Professor Kuo says you get small, but persistent benefits from even low doses of green space immersion – for example, just living in a tree-lined street and gazing at green views. But perhaps the greatest benefits come from my favourite pastime: walking in the woods.

So get outside into a park or a patch of woodland whenever you get the chance.

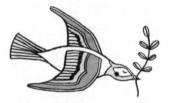

It is great to just stop, look around, breathe in the smell of the trees and appreciate the pattern of light passing through the leaves. Pausing to notice your environment in this way shifts your focus outwards, makes you more engaged in the world around you and less in your own thoughts.

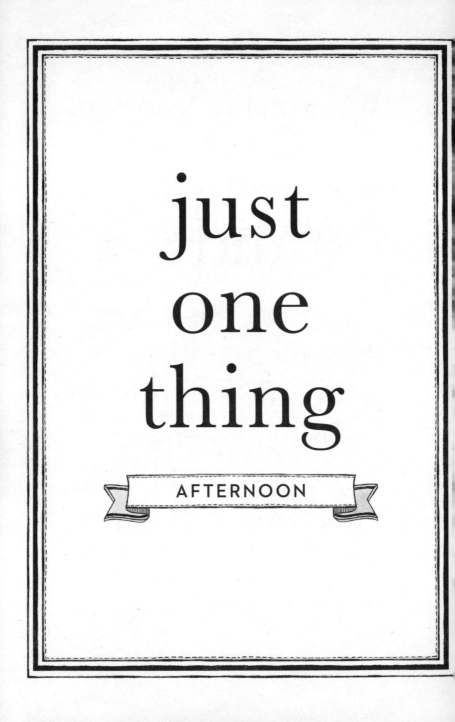

just one thing

AFTERNOON

stand up

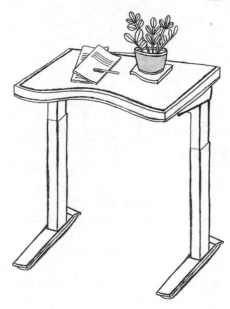

How to do it: stand up for two to three minutes every hour.

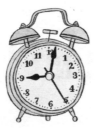

If you are a desk-based worker, as so many of us are, then by late afternoon you will have spent a lot of time sitting down, which is really bad for your body. Fortunately, there's a simple solution: standing up! Spending more time standing is good for your blood sugars and for your bones. It could even improve your psychological health.

We have known for a long time that lots of sitting, particularly when done in one long block, is bad for us. Back in the 1950s, researchers highlighted a stark difference in health between bus drivers (who sit all day) and bus conductors (who used to stand at the back of the bus, giving out tickets). They found the drivers were twice as likely to have heart attacks as the conductors.

Since then, plenty of studies have shown a sedentary lifestyle increases your risk of type 2 diabetes, heart disease, ageing generally and death from all causes.

Yet studies show that many of us spend 10 hours or more a day on our bottoms. If you drive for a living, your choices might be limited, but if your job or lifestyle allows, try to stand as much as possible – it really can make a big difference, both physically and mentally.

John Buckley, professor of applied exercise science at University Centre, Shrewsbury, told me that when we sit for long periods our bodies go into 'sleep' mode, shutting down many of the important functions that keep us healthy. 'As hunter-gatherers we were designed to be moving most of the day,' he says. 'Sitting slows our metabolism and drops everything to a resting level.

'However, when you stand up, all your systems function optimally, and gravity pulls your body without you realising – this small but constant force helps us to maintain muscle strength and bone density too.'

It seems our bodies need the constant, almost imperceptible increase in muscle activity that standing provides. The very simplest movement helps us to keep our all-important blood sugar under control.

You might hope you can offset the evils of spending all day on your bottom with a sweaty trip to the gym after work, but emerging evidence suggests that, unless you're doing 40 minutes of moderately vigorous exercise every single day, you cannot undo the damage that sitting causes. And even worse, if you sit for long periods each day you could be decreasing the benefits of any exercise you do.

The answer lies in taking the opportunity to stand whenever you can throughout your day and getting into the habit of spending more time on your feet than on your bottom.

STANDING TIPS

★ Invest in a standing desk. A recent trial found that, after 12 months of using a standing desk, volunteers reported feeling less anxious, less fatigued and better engaged with their work.

★ Set a ping alarm on your phone to remind you to stand up briefly every 30 minutes.

★ When the phone rings, stand up to take the call (better still, walk and talk).

★ Initiate 'standing meetings' or 'walking meetings'.

★ Stand on public transport.

★ Put the remote control out of reach so you have to get up every time you want to change channels.

★ Stand up at every TV advertisement break and do some stretches or squats.

CASE STUDY

Jake, communities manager

'I used to spend 99 per cent of my day sitting, in fact, I'd barely move at all other than at lunchtime, so it was a big change when Dr Mosley asked me to make a point of standing up every hour. One thing I did was arrange standing meetings with my colleagues, and I found I did feel more engaged. Then I started to naturally stand up to take phone calls. It really does make me feel more productive. Normally I'd get home and spend the evening sitting in front of the TV, but after standing at intervals throughout the day I feel more energised – this is an easy habit to make!'

As hunter-gatherers
we were designed
to be moving most
of the day. Sitting
slows our metabolism
and drops everything
to a resting level.

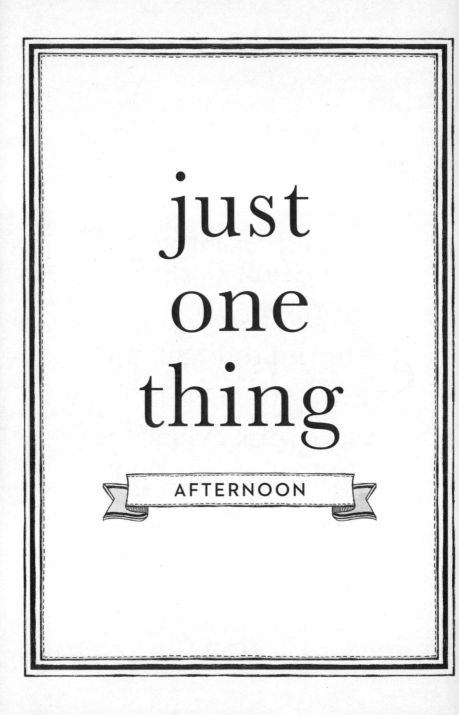

just
one
thing

AFTERNOON

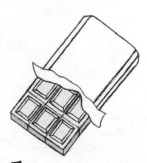

eat chocolate

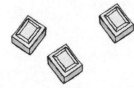

How to do it: replace sweet treats with a couple of squares of dark chocolate.

I have a seriously sweet tooth and the only way I can avoid unrestrained eating is to make sure there are no treats – and certainly no milk chocolate in the house. But I often allow myself a late-afternoon – or post-dinner-time treat – of a couple of small squares of dark chocolate. It helps satisfy my cravings for something sweet, while at the same time offering potential health benefits, such as lowering my blood pressure and even boosting my brain.

The health benefits of dark chocolate come from compounds called flavanols which we encountered earlier in apples. Flavanols are also present in cocoa beans – the darker the chocolate, the more flavanols it usually contains. Sadly, there are no flavanols in white chocolate and very few in milk chocolate, which I much prefer. With white and milk chocolate, the manufacturers process out the bitter-tasting cacao, adding sugar and milk to make it more palatable, but it is precisely those bitter compounds that have the health benefits.

Professor Aedin Cassidy is director of interdisciplinary research at Queens University Belfast and an expert on chocolate. She told me that one reason she eats dark chocolate regularly is that 'trials consistently show benefits and improvements in blood pressure, blood flow, insulin and cholesterol levels'.

Researchers first made the connection between cocoa and health when population studies involving indigenous people in Panama showed that their blood pressure did not increase with age as it does in many other parts of the world. This, they surmised, was due to the large quantities of unsweetened cocoa the Guna people typically drink (up to five cups a day).

More recently, a randomised controlled trial carried out in Germany and published in the *Journal of the American Medical Association* showed that eating dark chocolate does indeed produce some modest benefits. In this study, 44 middle-aged adults with high blood pressure were randomly allocated to either eating 6g of dark chocolate (two small squares) or 6g of white chocolate every evening for 18 weeks.

At the end of the study, only those who had been eating the dark chocolate saw improvements in their blood pressure, which dropped by an average of 3mmHg. That doesn't sound much but it was enough to reduce rates of hypertension in this group from 86 per cent to 68 per cent.

So how can dark chocolate be good for us? Well, it's partly because, as in the case of beetroot (see page 118), eating dark chocolate leads to the production of nitric oxide, which causes blood vessels to expand and consequently improve blood flow. But Professor Cassidy also believes that the flavanols in dark chocolate can 'feed' the 'good' bacteria that live in our gut.

'One of the most fascinating new areas of research is the impact of the gut on other aspects of our mental and physical health,' she told me. 'When you eat dark chocolate, it seems the flavanols reach all the way to the large intestine before being metabolised. There, gut bacteria munch them up and convert them into special compounds which then travel to the heart and brain. It is these compounds that appear to have the potential to produce protective effects – they seem to be able to boost cerebral blood flow, which aids learning and memory.'

Professor Cassidy recommends picking a dark chocolate with around 50 per cent cocoa solids – this is a compromise between very high cocoa solids (which can be very bitter) and low cocoa solids (which might be calorific and too tempting to indulge in).

CASE STUDY
Christine, a busy manager in the health service
Christine is normally surrounded by sweet treats, which she and other medics rely on to keep them going through long shifts. I asked her to ignore the cake and donuts and instead eat two squares of dark chocolate every time she felt the urge to reach for something sweet. She was delighted to accept the challenge: 'I'm really enjoying this experiment!' she says. 'I'm getting used to the taste of dark chocolate – it is difficult to stick to just two squares, but I do find that is enough to give me a boost if I'm about to take on a difficult task. In fact, I've been surprised at how well just two squares can get me through the afternoon energy slump and keep me going through to the evening.'

THE DARKER THE BETTER
The more cocoa solids a chocolate product contains, the more antioxidants it tends to contribute.

20g of dark chocolate (60% cocoa solids) contains 34mg of flavanols
20g of milk chocolate contains 14mg of flavanols
20g of white chocolate contains no flavanols

Researchers first made the connection between cocoa and health when population studies involving indigenous people in Panama showed that their blood pressure did not increase with age as it does in many other parts of the world.

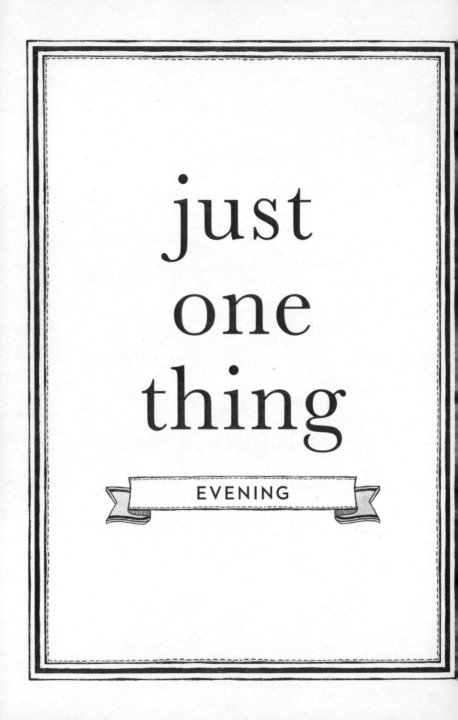

just one thing

EVENING

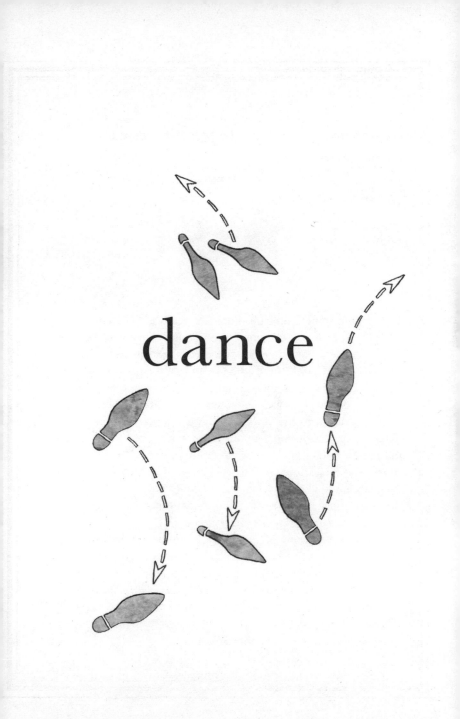

dance

How to do it: spend five to ten minutes dancing to music each day.

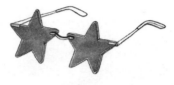

If you fancy something a bit more physically active than gaming, what about taking up dancing? I'm not one of the world's most natural movers, but I do enjoy the occasional evening of salsa with my wife, Clare. And if you like to bust out a few moves you will be pleased to hear that dancing, and trying out new routines, has been shown to be more effective than traditional fitness exercises for improving your muscles, balance and brain health. Dancing vigorously can get your heartbeat up to over 140 beats per minute and offers you a great combination of low- and high-intensity exercise bouts in the process.

In addition, dancing has been shown to help to alleviate depression, reduce your risk of heart disease and stroke, boost your memory and protect against dementia.

And the great thing is you don't have to be any good. Dr Julia Christensen from the Max Planck Institute in Germany, a former dancer who retrained as a neuroscientist, told me that competitive dancers are often very stressed when they are performing, while actually the key to getting the benefits from dancing is to be relaxed. So just enjoy yourself and dance as if no one else is watching (which they probably aren't).

Dr Christensen says dancing enhances all the known benefits of listening to music, by adding a social aspect. Because it encourages group cohesion and bonding, it appears to have a more powerful stress-reducing effect than merely listening to music.

It also seems to improve attention and helps us to be better at multitasking and planning.

Brain imaging studies have shown that dancing can increase the volume of the hippocampus (an area of the brain that deals with spatial memory) and improve white matter (the number of nerve cells) in areas of the brain associated with processing speed and memory.

Some of Dr Christensen's most fascinating research is looking into the science of 'interoception', the awareness of bodily feelings: 'By putting tiny electrodes on their fingers, we were able to show that people who dance are better able to recognise emotions in other people – their bodies actually react differently to emotional expressions.'

Apparently, we are all (even me!) natural dancers! 'Humans are the only species with a specific connection between ear and leg, which means we are hardwired to tune into the rhythm of our movements,' she says.

Dancing together is obviously more fun than dancing alone and may also help us manage pain because dancing enthusiastically with others triggers the release of endorphins, powerful hormones that can relieve pain and induce positive feelings.

The best thing to do is to join a weekly class. That will make you more likely to stick to it. Or you could sign up for some online classes to get you started at home. There is plenty to be gained from a bit of shimmying around the kitchen, or strutting your stuff in the bedroom.

I think dancing really is one of the best ways to keep your body and mind fit and healthy. It relieves stress, it's a workout and fundamentally: it feels great.

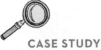

CASE STUDY

Lorne, travel company owner from Edinburgh

'The last time I did any dancing was when I won a disco competition at school – but that was a VERY long time ago! But I spent a week doing a little bit of dancing each morning with my children. It can feel a bit daft at times, with me boogying while everyone is rushing to grab breakfast and get out of the house but it's fun and it makes such a great start to the day – it definitely lifts my mood. I'm even doing an online dance class now – this could lead to a new exercise routine for me.'

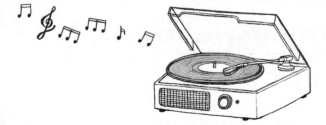

Apparently, we are all (even me!) natural dancers! Humans are the only species with a specific connection between ear and leg, which means we are hardwired to tune into the rhythm of our movements.

just
one
thing

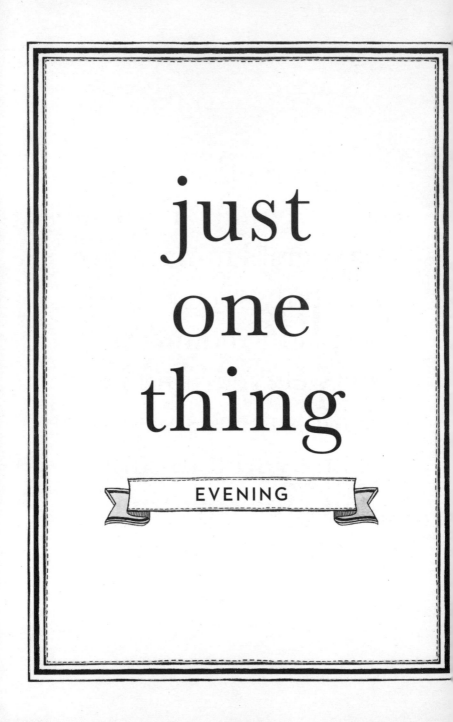

EVENING

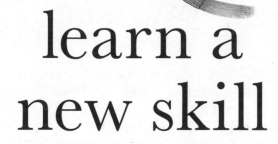

learn a
new skill

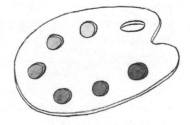

How to do it: pick something you find enjoyable and challenging, and devote 20–30 minutes to it each day.

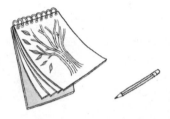

I recently had a go at painting. It was the first time I had tried to draw anything since I was a child, and the first time I had ever worked with oils. When the model came in and draped herself on a chair, I was terrified. I had no idea where to start.

The art teacher taught us the basics of perspective and how to mix oils, then left us to get on with it. I was there for a couple of hours, and I was surprised by how engrossing it was. I got the model's hands completely wrong, and her feet ended up as ugly pink blobs, but I was quietly pleased with the end result. And I want to go back.

Taking up video games, learning to dance or trying to paint are all very challenging, particularly when you are my age (65), but it is precisely because they are challenging that doing them has such a powerful effect on the ageing brain. As the US president John F Kennedy said, when launching the American race to the moon, 'We choose to go to the Moon in this decade and do the other things, not because they are easy, but because they are hard.'

It is a sentiment that Alan Gow, who is professor of psychology at Heriot-Watt University, would agree with. His research has shown that trying to acquire new skills later in life will not only give your brain a good workout, but may even mean you generate new brain cells.

'The evidence is suggesting it is possible to make changes you wouldn't have thought possible a few decades ago,' he says.

You might think that learning to play the piano, master Mandarin or get your head around the complexities of spreadsheets might be inherently stressful, but studies show the act of learning can actually reduce your stress levels.

In one study, volunteers were asked either to learn something new, or to do something relaxing. Perhaps surprisingly, it was the group learning new skills who saw the biggest reductions in levels of stress.

That's because when you are doing something that absorbs you, the outside world is put on hold. Like practising mindfulness, it effectively calms the critical voice in your head, which so often makes you focus on past failure and puts you down. The process of approaching something new, particularly when it is being done in a group with others, actually makes you less judgmental of your actions, and less stressed.

Learning something new can also change the way you think, as well as the way you feel. If the skill is challenging enough, your brain will be forced to forge new pathways and grow new connections, and this can quite literally boost your brain power.

Professor Gow's ongoing studies indicate that, after three months of working at a new skill, people show improvements in thinking skills – specifically in the areas of the brain most affected by the ageing process.

'Processing and thinking speeds tend to be among the first areas of brain function to start to decline with age, but we believe it is precisely these areas of brain function that most benefit from learning a new skill,' he explains.

'We believe it can reverse that feeling of "slowing down" you get with age, and if you continue mastering the skill, this benefit could extend to other thinking skills and improve memory too.'

So, thankfully, it seems you can teach an old dog new tricks. As Professor Gow says: 'It's never too late to try new things and the longer you stick at them, the more benefit you will accumulate over time.

'And people who maintain their thinking skills,' he adds, 'generally live longer, healthier lives – so it makes sense to embrace the chance to improve them.'

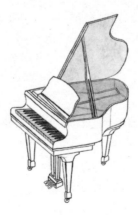

LEARN A LANGUAGE

One of the best things you can do for your brain is learn a new language, because that juggling between different sounds, words, concepts and grammatical and social rules enhances blood flow and connections across the entire brain. It can literally change your brain, boosting the number of brain cells and the connections between them. It can even improve your intelligence. But for maximum benefit, you have to throw yourself into the task and practise your new language for five hours a week!

WILL PUZZLES, CROSSWORDS AND SUDOKU HELP TRAIN THE BRAIN?

According to Professor Gow, solving complex sudoku puzzles or doing crosswords will help a bit, but these are nothing like as effective at preserving thinking skills as learning a new skill, such as dancing or painting.

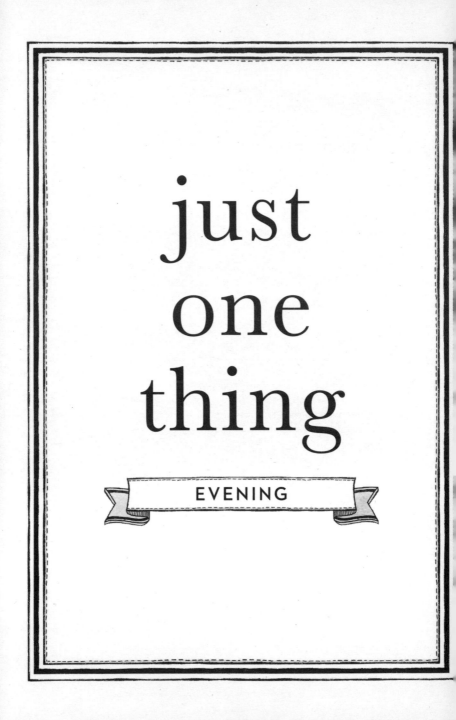

just one thing

EVENING

hot bath

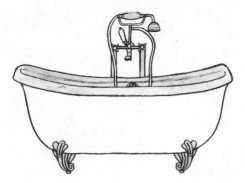

How to do it: enjoy a soak in a hot bath 90 minutes before bed.

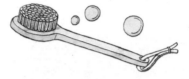

A deliciously relaxing hot bath is one of those rare pleasures in life that not only feels great but is actually good for you! Studies suggest that regular hot baths could help reduce blood sugar levels and lower your risk of heart disease. And those of you who struggle to drop off at night might like to know that a hot bath, taken an hour and a half before bedtime, could help you get to sleep quicker and improve the quality of your sleep.

Jason Ellis is professor of psychology at Northumbria University and director of the Northumbria Sleep Centre. He likes to have a hot bath at night and told me that one of the main reasons it helps promote sleep is because of the effect it has on your core body temperature. But you have to get the timing right.

When you have the hot bath your core body temperature goes up. But it is when you get out, and start to cool down, that you get the sleep-inducing benefits.

'As your core temperature falls, it mimics the onset of sleep, triggering the release of the sleep hormone, melatonin, and sending a strong signal that it is time for bed. There's a psychological impact, too,' he adds. 'A soak in the bath is valuable "me" time if you've had a busy day.'

Although he says a hot shower can work in a similar way, a bath is best – 'because you are fully immersing yourself in the hot water' – and he recommends aiming for a temperature of 40–42 degrees Celsius, around 90 minutes before bed, for maximum beneficial effect.

BOOST YOUR BATH BENEFITS

★ Dim the lights (darkness helps to boost melatonin, which triggers sleep).

★ Use lavender essential oil in the bath (studies show that inhaling it can improve sleep).

★ Put on some soft background music (studies show that classical music can improve sleep quality).

★ Instil a post-bath screen ban – no phone-scrolling (the stimulus plus blue light from any screen can make you feel alert and delay sleep onset).

Jen, mum of two and assistant practitioner in mental health
'I don't sleep very well and I've always found it hard to relax, but after a hot bath I did become really quite sleepy, and I slept better than I had in a long time. I noticed I had more energy the next day too. I've got into the habit of having a hot bath before bed three times a week and I'd definitely recommend this for anyone who struggles with their sleep.'

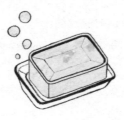

As your core temperature falls, it mimics the onset of sleep, triggering the release of the sleep hormone, melatonin, and sending a strong signal that it is time for bed.

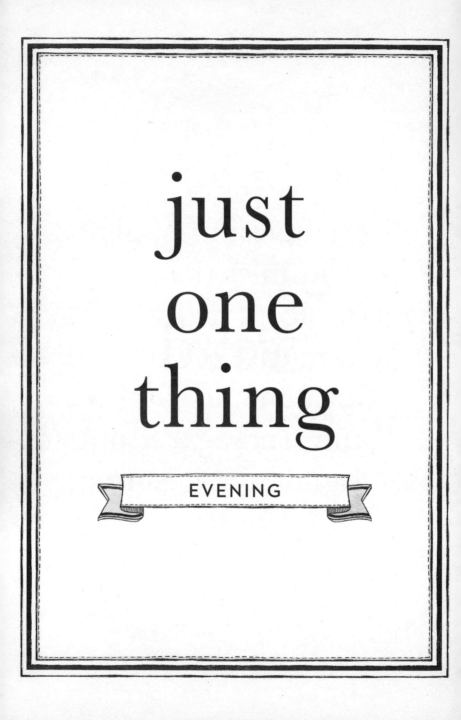

just one thing

EVENING

read

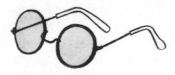

How to do it: read a book for 30 minutes each day, ideally a work of fiction.

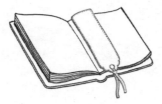

I absolutely love reading and have from a young age. I was often spotted walking down the street, reading avidly while trying to avoid fellow pedestrians and lamp posts. These days I snatch my reading moments when I can, such as during a lunch break, on a train or late at night. I'm also a member of a local book club, which over the past 10 years has provided a great deal of entertainment and food for thought, so I don't need any persuading that reading lots of fiction is good for empathy and social skills. Nor that it can help improve memory and protect against depression.

The great thing about reading fiction in particular is that it acts as a 'whole brain' workout. When researchers at Stanford University scanned the brains of people while they were reading Jane Austen (one of my favourite authors), they found a dramatic and unexpected increase in blood flow across the entire brain.

That's because when we get really immersed in a good book, our brains are busy imagining the settings, sounds, smells and tastes described, and this activates the many different areas of the brain that process these experiences in real life. Words like 'lavender', 'cinnamon' and 'soap', for example, will elicit a response not only in the language-processing areas of our brains, but also in the areas devoted to dealing with smells.

According to neuroscientist Dr Raymond Mar, at York University in Toronto, reading fiction can boost your empathy and interpersonal skills because the parts of the brain that we use to understand stories overlap with the ones we use to understand other people. 'Reading helps our brains get better at creating accurate models of real people and predicting what they might think, feel or do,' he told me.

I've always used books as a form of escapism, so I was not surprised to learn that studies show reading is one of the best ways to escape from the pressures of modern life. It is this aspect of reading that may reduce an avid reader's risk of developing depression.

'Anxiety is all about having attention focused inwardly,' says Dr Mar, 'but reading forces our focus on the words and the story and this can take us out of our head and help us to relax. We can enter a meditative state when we are really absorbed.'

Meanwhile, more remarkably, studies have shown that being a keen reader is also associated with a longer life, though I suspect this has a lot to do with the fact that people who read are also more likely to follow a healthier lifestyle. Research from Yale University found that those who read for 30 minutes a day lived on average 23 months longer than those who did not – the opposite of what happens if you spend the same amount of time watching TV.

So what should we be reading? Dr Mar favours novels or biographies (as opposed to non-fiction). The key thing is that the reader finds themselves immersed in a story. 'It's important you find something you enjoy reading,' he says, pointing out that the positive benefits occur only after repeated, long-term and frequent exposure.

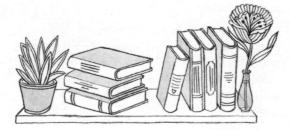

Reading fiction in particular acts as a 'whole brain' workout. When researchers at Stanford University scanned the brains of people while they were reading Jane Austen, they found a dramatic and unexpected increase in blood flow across the entire brain.

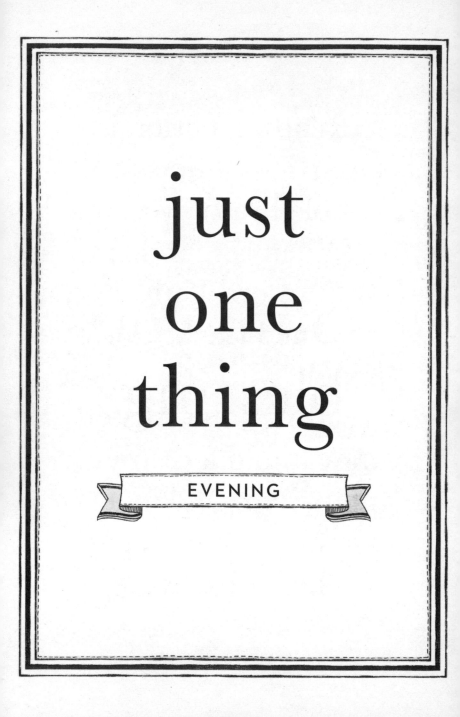

just one thing

EVENING

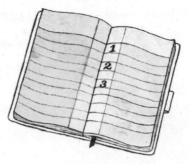

count your
blessings

How to do it: last thing at night before bed, write down three things for which you feel grateful.

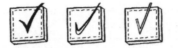

The idea that you should 'count your blessings' might sound a bit old-fashioned, but there is solid science behind the claims that getting into the habit of being regularly grateful not only makes you feel happier, but can also lower your blood pressure, improve your sleep, ease pain and even rewire your brain, with lasting effects. How can something so simple be so powerful? And how can you access it?

According to Dr Fuschia Sirois, a psychology professor at Durham University who specialises in investigating gratitude, self-compassion and their role in health and wellbeing, 'One of the simplest ways is to think about three things for which you can be grateful that day. Perhaps someone has acted kindly towards you, or perhaps you noticed it was a bright sunny day, or you had the opportunity to get outside and enjoy the fresh air.'

The aim of regular gratitude practice is to develop what she calls a 'grateful mindset' which can have powerfully positive effects.

'There are lots of different theories about how gratitude works,' she told me. 'Perhaps gratitude puts you in a more positive state, opens up your perspective, allowing you to focus on and appreciate the positive instead of focusing on your worries. If you have trouble sleeping, this can certainly help.

'We have found that gratitude can reduce stress levels by helping us to see things from a broader perspective, rather than via the narrow view we tend to adopt when our fight and flight mechanisms are activated,' she adds.

'If gratitude can down-regulate our stress response, it makes sense that it could have a positive influence on contributing mechanisms such as inflammation, which is a risk marker for a number of different chronic diseases.'

Professor Sirois and her team have been studying the benefits of gratitude for people living in ongoing stressful situations, such as those with chronic health conditions. In their trial, the participants who spent three weeks counting their blessings reported significantly less pain, as well as better sleep, than those in the control group.

She thinks this could be because pain perception can be easily amplified by stress and negative feelings, and if expressing gratitude can ease those negative feelings, then the extent to which you feel pain can be affected too.

Other research shows that a grateful mindset can increase the chance that you might adopt healthy habits (eating healthily and exercising regularly, for instance), and has identified a link the researchers refer to as 'future orientation' (the extent to which an individual thinks about the future and anticipates future consequences).

One American study found that asking people to write a 'gratitude list' resulted in higher rates of happiness and less physical illness. After two months of journalling, the participants also began doing more exercise, perhaps because they were feeling better about life.

'When you look at research about the neurological changes that happen in the brains of people who tend to be grateful, you can see that areas in the brain that are activated when people experience gratitude tend to be the same areas that are linked with the capacity to think about the future outcomes of their actions,' Professor Sirois says.

So adopting a grateful mindset can help to shift your thought processes from negative to positive and the feelgood chemicals that are released may even help to rewire your brain.

I should point out that not all research into gratitude journalling has produced glowing results and if you have serious concerns about your mental health you should talk to your GP. But if, like me, you are someone who occasionally tends to dwell on the dark side of life, counting your blessings and writing them down might really help.

And that feels like a good place to end. So let me finish by saying that making the podcast series Just One Thing is one of the best things I've done, and I'm truly grateful to all the people who contributed to the series and to this book. I do hope you've enjoyed reading it and that you give Just One Thing a go...

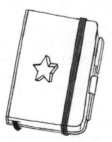

TIPS FOR EFFECTIVE GRATITUDE JOURNALLING

★ Keep a notebook and pen by your bed.

★ Allocate 15 minutes to writing in it at night every night.

★ Just jot down in note form three things that you are thankful for.

★ Has someone showed you kindness?

★ What small things made you feel good today?

★ Is there someone in your life you are grateful for? Why?

★ What skills or abilities are you thankful to have?

★ What elements of nature are you grateful for and why?

CASE STUDY
Nathan, fitness instructor
'I was asked to sit down at bedtime each evening and write down three things I'm grateful for, but within a few nights I found I was just too tired when I got to bed to focus properly. So instead I decided to make it something I'd do each morning when I woke up. I found this a great way to start the day and I've been surprised at how easy it is to find things to be grateful for. I think this exercise forces you to think about what makes you happy; it makes you appreciate what you have, and it broadens your mindset. In fact, I'd say I'm very grateful I've got the opportunity to practise gratitude journalling!'

ENDNOTES

INTRODUCTION
https://onlinelibrary.wiley.com/doi/abs/10.1002/ejsp.674

CH 1 EARLY MORNING

Intelligent exercises
(1) https://www.health.harvard.edu/staying-healthy/more-push-ups-may-mean-less-risk-of-heart-problems
(2) https://pubmed.ncbi.nlm.nih.gov/31216005/

Cold shower
(1) https://pubmed.ncbi.nlm.nih.gov/8925815/
(2) https://www.ncbi.nlm.nih.gov/pmc/articles/PMC2211456/
(3) https://www.ncbi.nlm.nih.gov/pmc/articles/PMC5025014/
(4) https://www.ncbi.nlm.nih.gov/pmc/articles/PMC7730683/shower

Sing
(1) https://www.ncbi.nlm.nih.gov/pmc/articles/PMC3860955/
(2) https://pubmed.ncbi.nlm.nih.gov/27515501/
(3) https://pubmed.ncbi.nlm.nih.gov/30534062/
(4) https://journals.sagepub.com/doi/abs/10.1177/13591053211012778

Meditate
(1) https://www.ncbi.nlm.nih.gov/pmc/articles/PMC3004979/
(2) https://jamanetwork.com/journals/jamainternalmedicine/fullarticle/2110998
(3) https://www.ncbi.nlm.nih.gov/pmc/articles/PMC5934947/
(4) https://pubmed.ncbi.nlm.nih.gov/24096366/
(5) https://news.harvard.edu/gazette/story/2018/04/harvard-researchers-study-how-mindfulness-may-change-the-brain-in-depressed-patients/
(6) https://www.health.harvard.edu/pain/mindfulness-meditation-to-control-pain
(7) https://www.ncbi.nlm.nih.gov/pmc/articles/PMC8430251/

Early-morning walk

(1) https://www.sleephealthjournal.org/article/S2352-7218(17)30041-4/
fulltext
(2) https://www.ulster.ac.uk/news/2018/june/study-finds-walking-
faster-could-help-you-live-longer

CH 2 BREAKFAST

Change your mealtimes

(1) https://pubmed.ncbi.nlm.nih.gov/22608008/
(2) https://www.surrey.ac.uk/news/many-people-could-reduce-their-
feeding-window-three-hours-finds-new-time-restricted-feeding-study
(3) https://www.salk.edu/news-release/clinical-study-finds-eating-within-
10-hour-window-may-help-stave-off-diabetes-heart-disease/

Drink water

(1) https://www.bda.uk.com/resource/the-importance-of-hydration.html
(2) https://www.alzdiscovery.org/cognitive-vitality/blog/can-dehydration-
impair-cognitive-function
(3) https://westminsterresearch.westminster.ac.uk/item/v7599/drinking-
water-enhances-cognitive-performance-positive-effects-on-working-
memory-but-not-long-term-memory
(4) https://pubmed.ncbi.nlm.nih.gov/26200171/
(5) http://pure-oai.bham.ac.uk/ws/portalfiles/portal/18685679/parretti_
waterpreloadingRCT.pdf

Eat some bacteria

(1) https://pubmed.ncbi.nlm.nih.gov/33693453/
(2) https://pubmed.ncbi.nlm.nih.gov/25998000/

Stand on one leg

(1) https://www.nature.com/articles/sj.bdj.2018.1062
(2) https://pubmed.ncbi.nlm.nih.gov/17503879/
(3) https://www.ncbi.nlm.nih.gov/pmc/articles/PMC6873344/
(4) https://www.bmj.com/content/348/bmj.g2219

Drink coffee

(1) https://www.bmj.com/content/359/bmj.j5024
(2) https://www.hsph.harvard.edu/news/hsph-in-the-news/coffee-depression-women-ascherio-lucas/
(3) https://www.nottingham.ac.uk/news/brown-fat-and-coffee
(4) https://aru.ac.uk/news/coffee-linked-to-lower-body-fat-in-women

CH 3 MID-MORNING

Take a break

(1) https://www.sciencedirect.com/science/article/pii/S0003687016302666
(2) https://www.nhm.ac.uk/discover/how-listening-to-bird-song-can-transform-our-mental-health.html
(3) https://www.ncbi.nlm.nih.gov/pmc/articles/PMC3779797/

Deep breaths

(1) https://www.ncbi.nlm.nih.gov/pmc/articles/PMC6137615/
(2) https://www.ncbi.nlm.nih.gov/pmc/articles/PMC5455070/
(3) https://pubmed.ncbi.nlm.nih.gov/30826382/
(4) https://pubmed.ncbi.nlm.nih.gov/21939499/

Exercise less, but more often

(1) https://journals.lww.com/acsm-msse/Fulltext/2019/06000/Association_between_Bout_Duration_of_Physical.16.aspx
(2) https://www.ncbi.nlm.nih.gov/pmc/articles/PMC4202748/

Eccentric exercise

(1) https://pubmed.ncbi.nlm.nih.gov/28291022/
(2) https://www.ncbi.nlm.nih.gov/pmc/articles/PMC6510035/

Think yourself stronger

(1) https://www.ncbi.nlm.nih.gov/pmc/articles/PMC6535038/
(2) https://bmcmedicine.biomedcentral.com/articles/10.1186/1741-7015-9-75

CH 4 LUNCHTIME

Enjoy oily fish

(1) https://www.sciencedaily.com/releases/2021/03/210308131709.htm
(2) https://www.ncbi.nlm.nih.gov/pmc/articles/PMC3917688/
(3) https://www.ncbi.nlm.nih.gov/pmc/articles/PMC4113767/
(4) https://www.ncbi.nlm.nih.gov/pmc/articles/PMC6683166/
(5) https://www.ncbi.nlm.nih.gov/pmc/articles/PMC4965662/
(6) https://pubmed.ncbi.nlm.nih.gov/34872587/

Eat beetroot

(1) https://www.ncbi.nlm.nih.gov/pmc/articles/PMC6515411/
(2) https://sshs.exeter.ac.uk/news/research/title_37371_en.html
(3) https://pubmed.ncbi.nlm.nih.gov/21471821/
(4) https://www.ncbi.nlm.nih.gov/pmc/articles/PMC6683255/
(5) https://academic.oup.com/jn/article/143/6/818/4571708?login=true

An apple a day

(1) https://pubmed.ncbi.nlm.nih.gov/22019438/
(2) https://pubmed.ncbi.nlm.nih.gov/29086478/
(3) https://www.cambridge.org/core/journals/british-journal-of-nutrition/article/apple-intake-is-inversely-associated-with-allcause-and-diseasespecific-mortality-in-elderly-women/EC7A2E4916E6A660649736CE42189685
(4) https://pubmed.ncbi.nlm.nih.gov/31584311/

Get some sun

(1) https://www.ed.ac.uk/news/2021/sunlight-linked-with-lower-covid-19-deaths
(2) https://www.ncbi.nlm.nih.gov/pmc/articles/PMC6013996/
(3) https://www.ncbi.nlm.nih.gov/pmc/articles/PMC1470481/
(4) https://www.ncbi.nlm.nih.gov/pmc/articles/PMC6490896/
(5) https://www.ed.ac.uk/news/2013/sunshine-080513

Take a nap

(1) https://www.bmj.com/company/newsroom/once-or-twice-weekly-daytime-nap-linked-to-lower-heart-attack-stroke-risk/
(2) https://news.berkeley.edu/2010/02/22/naps_boost_learning_capacity/
(3) https://news.mit.edu/2021/india-sleep-study-economics-0729

CH 5 AFTERNOON

Get some house plants

(1) https://www.lung.org/clean-air/at-home/indoor-air-pollutants/volatile-organic-compounds#:~:text=VOCs%20Can%20Harm%20Health,effects%2C%20though%20many%20have%20several.
(2) https://link.springer.com/article/10.1007/s11270-006-9124-z

Play video games

(1) https://www.jstor.org/stable/27032854
(2) https://www.psychologicalscience.org/news/releases/2020-sept-violent-video-games.html
(3) https://www.ncbi.nlm.nih.gov/pmc/articles/PMC2921999/

Green spaces

(1) https://www.ncbi.nlm.nih.gov/pmc/articles/PMC7913501/
(2) https://www.ncbi.nlm.nih.gov/pmc/articles/PMC8408569/
(3) https://www.nature.com/articles/s41893-021-00781-9
(4) https://www.ncbi.nlm.nih.gov/pmc/articles/PMC4548093/
(5) https://www.tandfonline.com/doi/full/10.1080/15622975.2021.1938670

Stand up

(1) http://www.epi.umn.edu/cvdepi/study-synopsis/london-transport-workers-study/
(2) https://evidence.nihr.ac.uk/alert/standing-desks-with-a-support-package-reduce-time-sitting-at-work/
(3) https://www.sciencealert.com/getting-a-sweat-on-for-30-40-minutes-could-offset-a-day-of-sitting-down

Eat chocolate
(1) https://www.ncbi.nlm.nih.gov/pmc/articles/PMC6478304/
(2) https://www.ncbi.nlm.nih.gov/pmc/articles/PMC5537860/
(3) https://www.birmingham.ac.uk/news/2020/can-drinking-cocoa-
make-you-smarter
(4) https://www.ncbi.nlm.nih.gov/pmc/articles/PMC4580960/
(5) https://www.nicswell.co.uk/health-news/does-eating-a-few-squares-
of-dark-chocolate-a-day-improve-blood-pressure
(6) https://www.ncbi.nlm.nih.gov/pmc/articles/PMC7071338/

6 EVENING

Dance
(1) https://www.ajpmonline.org/article/S0749-3797(16)00030-1/fulltext
(2) https://www.frontiersin.org/articles/10.3389/fpsyg.2019.00936/full
(3) https://www.coventry.ac.uk/primary-news/salsa-dancing-boosts-
brain-function-says-coventry-university-study-for-tv-show/
(4) https://depts.washington.edu/mbwc/news/article/dancing-
to-remember
(5) https://www.frontiersin.org/articles/10.3389/fnhum.2017.00305/full
(6) https://www.ox.ac.uk/news/2015-10-28-dancing-raises-pain-threshold'

Learn a new skill
(1) https://michiganross.umich.edu/rtia-articles/study-learning-something-
new-could-help-reduce-stress
(2) https://www.ncbi.nlm.nih.gov/pmc/articles/PMC5065201/

Hot bath
(1) https://www.lboro.ac.uk/news-events/news/2018/november/hot-
baths-help-metabolism-and-inflammation/
(2) https://www.ncbi.nlm.nih.gov/pmc/articles/PMC5023696/
(3) https://www.sciencedirect.com/science/article/abs/pii/
S1087079218301552?via%3Dihub
(4) https://pubmed.ncbi.nlm.nih.gov/24720812/
(5) https://pubmed.ncbi.nlm.nih.gov/18426457/

Read

(1) https://news.stanford.edu/news/2012/september/austen-reading-fmri-090712.html
(2) https://jamanetwork.com/journals/jamapsychiatry/article-abstract/2681169
(3) https://www.ncbi.nlm.nih.gov/books/NBK453237/
(4) https://yalealumnimagazine.com/articles/4377-bookworms-live-longer

Count your blessings

(1) https://greatergood.berkeley.edu/article/item/how_gratitude_changes_you_and_your_brain
(2) https://www.sciencedirect.com/science/article/abs/pii/S0022399920301847

First published in Great Britain in 2022 by
Short Books, an imprint of
Octopus Publishing Group Limited
Carmelite House
50 Victoria Embankment
London
EC4Y 0DZ

An Hachette UK Company
www.hachette.co.uk
www.octopusbooks.co.uk

This paperback edition first published in 2023

By arrangement with BBC Studios Productions.
The BBC and BBC Studios logos are trademarks of the
British Broadcasting Corporation and are used under licence.
BBC and BBC Studios logos © British Broadcasting Corporation.

Distributed in the US by
Hachette Book Group
1290 Avenue of the Americas
4th and 5th Floors
New York, NY 10104

Cover design: Mel Four
Text design: Smith & Gilmour
Illustration: Lindsey Spinks
Production: Emily Noto

ISBN: 978-1-78072-590-1

A CIP catalogue record for this book is available from the British Library.

Printed and bound in Great Britain by Clays Ltd, Elcograf S.p.A

13

This FSC® label means that materials used for the product have been
responsibly sourced.

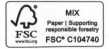

MIX
Paper | Supporting
responsible forestry
FSC® C104740